Edward Miskie's

CANCER,
Musical Theatre
& OTHER
CHRONIC ILLNESSES

10-Year Cancer Survivorship Edition

Cancer, Musical Theatre & Other Chronic Illnesses: 10-Year Cancer Survivorship Anniversary Edition

Original publication via KDP © 2017 Edward Miskie

ISBN 9798986539393 (hardcover)
ISBN 9798987044704 (paperback)
ISBN 9798987044728 (eBook)

Title Credit: Alex Peariman
Cover Photo: Lauren Althea
Cover Design: Edward Miskie
Editing, Formatting & Layout Design: Megs Thompson

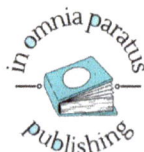

www.inomniaparatuspublishing.com

Edward Miskie's

CANCER,
Musical Theatre
& OTHER
CHRONIC ILLNESSES

10-Year Cancer Survivorship Edition

This book is for Steven LoCasicio, Alex Fleicher, and Nellie Horetsky: The beautiful humans in my life who helped inspire and write this book.

To Donnie Long, Brandon Stamm, Grandpa Bob, and Grandpa John who may not be physically with us but are still with us.

My friends, my heart; Alex, Vanessa, Murj, Brandon, Greg, Rayne, Bobby, Brooke, Barbara, Bosco, Badiene, Sarah, Taylor, Mary, Gabriel, Berto, Michael Huns, Kristen, Ryan, Jordan, Scarlet, Jerami, Amanda, Gloria, Roger, Ruthann, Craig and Ariela, everyone at Sloan-Kettering - Emily - and everyone who contributed to ThereAreGiants, BariToned, and Edward the First. You all kept me going and alive in some way if not literally, and for that I am eternally grateful.

To Megs for making this re-publication possible.

And especially, and most importantly my family - Mom, Dad, Madeline, Monica, Grandma Betty, Grandma Jan, Aunt Del - who without fail support and encourage and guide me in ways I can't even express.

Thank you all for the last ten years of my life.

Here's to ten more!

Table of Contents

Preface

August 2022

Divorced, Beheaded, Survived!

Not to state the obvious, but I am not directly associated with the Broadway smash hit musical SIX. I am not *in* the Broadway smash hit musical SIX, nor am I one of the fabulous wives of Henry VIII in the Broadway smash hit musical SIX. But I have divorced myself, beheaded the person I was before, and somehow survived to tell the tale. So, when I say that I have a loose understanding of what being victimized by the original Regina George is like... I'm lying. I don't. But after spending DAYS binge-listening to the songs of the Broadway smash hit musical SIX, I knew I wanted to use it as the theme to reintroduce this, the 10-Year Cancer Survivorship Anniversary Re-Published Edition of my book. I couldn't help myself, and trust me, you'll thank me later. Regardless of whether this is my backwards attempt to find a place within this phenomenal, all-woman presenting show, there is actually a tie-in, a method to my madness. I just haven't shared it yet.

If Henry VIII is cancer, which let's face it, he was, and each of his wives was a stage of who you were then, and are now, I could arguably say that to achieve Kathryn Parr status of survivor, you'd first need to travel through the often bloody and unbecoming Aragon's and Boleyn's to get there. I don't mean literally of course, queen, but hear me out, I mean, you're already here, so what've you got to lose? Your head?

Divorced.

Despite that I reference having a traumatic break-up in this book, that's not what I'm referring to when I talk about my divorce. By divorce, I mean from myself. From my old self. From the self I was before I was diagnosed, and the self I was when I was told I was cancer free. I cut her off. Stopped paying her bills and stopped letting her live rent free inside my head. I am no longer that bitch, and

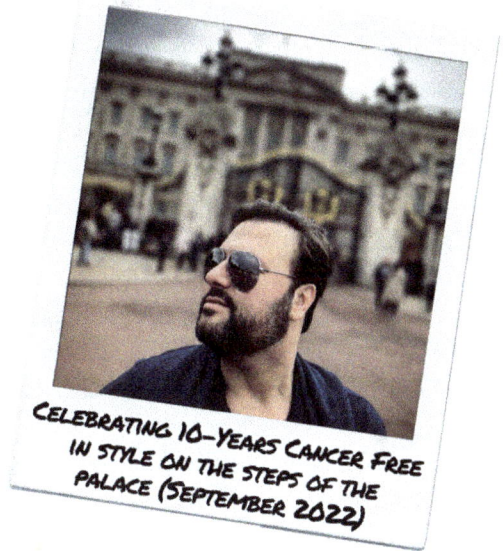

CELEBRATING 10-YEARS CANCER FREE IN STYLE ON THE STEPS OF THE PALACE (SEPTEMBER 2022)

that's okay. That's actually wonderfully okay. Who needs that lowbrow anyway? Without her hanging around, I was able to move on, grow, and sparkle. I'm free. Not just free from hospitals and chemo, but free from a life I mistakenly believed was going to bring me happiness. Free from a life that's no longer mine; that no longer exists. Free.

Sounds incredible, huh? Liberating? Scary? Well, honestly being scared was the best part. Scared meant I cared. Scared meant I was doing something new, exciting, and unfamiliar. Scared meant I was already growing!

So, how does one accomplish this divorce? Well, how does one accomplish any divorce? I had to make the decision that I was done. Done trying to keep my relationship with my former self alive. I reached the point where I knew it was over, that I wanted something more. I saw a different future for myself. I wanted out!

Living in trauma does one thing – it holds you back. Making that trauma your identity does one thing – it holds you back.

By divorcing myself from that moment in my life, I was able to recognize that it happened, move on to accept the things I learned from the experience, and walk away. It was the best thing I've ever done. Just like every other kind of divorce!

Now, just like every other kind of divorce, this one was messy. It wasn't cut and dry. It wasn't fun, and it definitely wasn't as simple as signing on the dotted line to separate assets. This divorce was titanic. The mental tap dancing I had to do to slay my way through the hyperbolic marriages I had fashioned with myself was a feat not even Fred Astaire would consider simple. I was forced to face and dismantle the marriage I held to an identity I created for myself while I was in the hospital as well as the marriages I held to excuses and stories I'd constructed to tell my friends, employers, coworkers, and myself about how I was doing.

"Psht! Fuck this cancer in the ass; I'm queen of the world and it won't win."

"I barely feel a thing and I'm going to keep living my life like nothing's happening."

Well, those paper machete façades can only stand so long, and eventually I had to tear them down page by page. It sucked, but oh my Katharine Parr was it worth it.

The marriages we let go of range from the physical – our former body, to the structural – our former goals and aspirations, and to marriages of the heart – relationships, friendships, and family. Like all divorces, no one loses everything.

To an extent, we're each afforded the opportunity to pick and choose what we'd like to take with us as we move onto the next chapter of our lives. This is, of course, not always the case, but for this scenario we're going to say that you have a choice of what you want to take with you.

Family, friends, and relationships are by far, the hardest of these three to divorce. I was extremely fortunate that I didn't have to cut any of my family off in the divorce, but there are plenty of scenarios where that could have happened had I not felt safe or taken care of during and after my treatments. So, when weighing this level of divorce, ask yourself – *Do I feel safe? Do I feel taken care of?* Friends and relationships will fluctuate, fall apart, and disappear entirely, but when the dust settles from those divorces, it's important to remember that what you're left with are the most valuable; the ones who will continue to stick by your side regardless of how bald, bloated, hormonal, or sickly you may be.

The best part about all of this marrying and divorcing myself business is that I got to ask myself with reckless abandon – reckless because after nearly dying what did I really have to lose anyway? *What do I want? Like, really, what do I want?* No holds barred. What is it that I want? I'm free now. I get to live. I get to go get it; What I want.

Beheaded.

As with the beheading of Anne Boleyn, it won't always be a single swift chop, the process may take a lot longer than you thought. You may even linger in a state of semi-decapitation, contemplating the final blow that'll eventually save you by killing off the host. But which do you keep? The head? Or the body? Do you have to make a choice? Since the only way to change your life is to change your mind… I recommend keeping the body. The body that will stumble around as the new head takes shape. Sure, it'll fall, and trip, and land in weird places and positions, but that's all a part of the learning and growth process.

In this scenario not only are you the beheaded, but your own executioner as well.

During chemo number two, I started to develop a pretty hefty drinking habit. It wasn't gradual. What can I say? When I do something, I do it all the way. It's been ten years, and I am only now really staring full sobriety in the face. The beheading is almost complete, but Annie B is still holding on by a spinal thread. She's a stubborn old broad.

The person I was before cancer? I don't know if I'd want to hang out with him today.

He was a know-it-all when in reality, he didn't know much at all. He was a little too big for his britches and looking for an easy win on every corner. He thought he was hot shit, and at the same time, thought he wasn't shit at all. He was deeply, deeply insecure - hungry for a glamorous future but without any desire to do the work required to build one. He didn't care too much about hurting or offending anyone and chalked it up to being "blunt" or just "saying what he was thinking." If we're being honest, he makes my skin crawl. Now don't get me wrong, he was hot as fuck, but at the time had no idea.

I think he's best summed up by a Marina and the Diamonds song lyric in which she says, *"I feel like I'm the worst, so I always act like I'm the best."*

Unironically, he loved that song.

Honestly, if I met that guy today, I'd gladly Anne Boleyn his ass. Cancer knocked him down several pegs: several, many pegs. And thank Marlow & Moss because that person, the pre-beheaded me, I'm nearly positive wouldn't have turned out to be very agreeable at all.

Now, I realize the ability to behead my former self with some ease was a privilege; I was single, I didn't have children, I didn't have a job, or much of a career to speak of. My living situation, albeit shady, was affordable and mostly simple. I was living an 'any way the wind blows' kind of life.

For most people, their beheading isn't quite so cut and dry. But you've got to do it. Unleash the guillotine. Not only because trying to recreate a person from the past in the present is nearly impossible, but because that person then becomes a cancer in-and-of themselves, within you.

Lower the blade and watch that head roll.

Survived.

Hang onto your heads! By 'survived' I don't really mean cancer. I mean life… after cancer.

Ten years ago, when I was told I was officially cancer free, I was shown an open window through which I was flung back into a pedestrian life that didn't include hospital routines, regiments, and guidance. It also didn't include a shred of an existence that I recognized. Where was I? Who was I? This should have been an exhilarating, exciting, and celebratory time for me. It seemed that way for everyone else. They were elated that I was no longer committed to chemo and cancer protocols. Everyone else was grateful for me, for my life, for my presence.

"I knew you'd pull through."

"If anyone was going to beat this, you were!"

"I'm so proud of you! You beat cancer."

Sure, those things all sound nice, but like... I didn't do anything. I showed up to my appointments and let my medical team do the work. If anything, I was self-sabotaging my survival by engaging in very risky, dangerous, and otherwise unhealthy behaviors and habits. Things weren't looking good, so there was a whole lot of "fuck it, let's do it" happening.

My entr'acte into life after cancer should have been the launch-pad from which I rocketed myself into a new, improved version of myself. In some ways, and eventually that's what I did. But through that window I also found that I was without a compass, without recognition, without... just without. This perpetuated my being mired with insecurities. Body insecurities, self-worth insecurities, life trajectory, and goal insecurities. Who was I? Where was I going? What did I want? Again, and again, and again.

Through that window I found myself asking "Ok, what do I do now?" I wasn't well enough to work, but I wasn't sick enough not to. I wasn't well enough to pursue relationships, or dating, or career goals, but I wasn't sick enough not to. So, what was I to do? I didn't know. I still don't know. But I had to do something, so, I flung shit in every direction in hopes that something would either stick or take off. I started serial dating, serial hooking-up, serial auditioning, serial content creation. Was I creating distractions so I wouldn't have to deal with other things? Maybe? Maybe. Probably. I was searching. That I know is true. I was searching because I was lost.

Survival mode often makes us default to what we know. Instinct. What I knew was gym, auditions, and menial jobs. So that's what I did. I'd wake up, go to the gym, honor the audition calendar I'd created for myself, and I'd go to work hocking t-shirts, and magnets at Broadway shows. I floated through the next year or so in this pattern. There are pictures of me from the time where I look dead behind the eyes. Unfeeling. Void. Because I was.

By 2017, five years after I was dubbed cancer free, my oncologist gave me a five-year pin and informed me that I was no longer going to be seeing her for yearly follow-ups. I cried. Which was *not* the reaction I anticipated. By 2017 I had completed ten contracts under which I performed all over the country. I'd also created and was performing my own concert, and I'd written and published this book the first time.

"OMG you're SO accomplished."

To the outsider? Yeah, sure. I've done a lot. A lot of which I am proud of. But a lot of what I've done was a desperate attempt to shed the routines and practices of being a full-time patient. To feel alive. To feel relevant. To feel part of something. Coping mechanisms. This book included. When I tried to turn *Cancer, Musical Theatre, and Other Chronic Illnesses* into an audiobook-slash-podcast, going back and reading or listening to these chapters was… fucking uncomfortable. There's a lot of headspace to navigate in association with the accomplishments, that I fully created myself. Guilty, but alive.

I guess so far, I've created a pretty bleak, sad-sack narrative of what surviving cancer is like. That wasn't really my intention. Life is good, simple and easy, or complicated and tough. So often we're shown the 'OMG you survived cancer: cue rainbows, glitter, and butterflies' version of this narrative, and that's simply not the reality. There's so much more below that surface, and that's what I set out to explore in this preface, this book, my story.

As far as MY survivorship journey. In the year 2022 I think I found my compass. It took me ten years of half-assed attempts, and to no one's surprise, only when I full-assed it, and TRIED, did I find my way.

A few updates for you:

- I left theatre to focus on TV, film, and voiceover.

- I pursued my adolescent aspirations of being a popstar and have created some music I'm pretty proud of. Check it out on all major streaming platforms under the name Edward the First.

- I'm producing a feature film called Ladylike written by the brilliant Taylor Coriell whom I am proud AF to call a friend.

- I'm producing some projects of my own with the brilliant Sarah Seeds whom I am also proud AF to call a friend. One of those projects is this book reimagined as a musical episodic TV show. Look out for that!

- I moved out of my 225 square foot studio apartment in the Upper West Side with a super shady rental agreement.

- I have my very own apartment, no strings, no agreements, that's way larger than the last one, albeit way more expensive, but it's mine and only mine.

- I have more agency over myself and my career than I ever have in the past and it feels amazing.

- My relationships with friends and family are stronger and more authentic than ever before.

- I'm mostly fully sober.

- I've been single for almost 9 years. Do I wish I had someone special in my life? Maybe. I don't know. For now, I'm good. Like, really good. I'm more stable than I've ever been. And if something comes along, well…we'll see.

- I co-parent a dog named Riley with a new neighbor in my building. She's a rescue, and I love her. She being the dog. The neighbor is not a rescue, but I do also love her.

- Things are pretty fabulous right now. I don't have any *real* complaints.

So, divorcing, beheading, and surviving is what worked for me. It's what I needed to do for myself. And, if my getting vulnerable and raw with you here helps you to stop watering dead plants, and feeding dead cats sooner than later, then by the head of Kathryn Howard, it's my pleasure.

The concept of divorced, beheaded, and survived is not just specific to cancer patients, or survivors either. Clearly, as it's a theme in the international musical theatre hit, SIX!! (I should be getting paid for show promo at this point. How many times have I mentioned that show now?) Anyone, and everyone can do this. It's going to look differently for each of us, as we're all different. But find whatever Henry VIII is holding you down or holding you back and move on. Do the hard thing. Do it now!

So, without further ado, take your seat, put your cell phone on silent, and get ready for the show of your life.

A-5, 6, 7, 8…

Edward Miskie

Act One

Edward Miskie

The Prologue

Cancer is really fucking terrible. I think we can all agree on some level that we know that. We've all seen, on either stage or screen, how cancer is portrayed; bald, and skinny with no appetite, tired. Mostly, that's all true...ish. My fellow patients and survivors understand. We know that the surface of all this patient business is just that: surface, but we don't stop being human; we don't stop feeling, needing, wanting. Maybe those of you

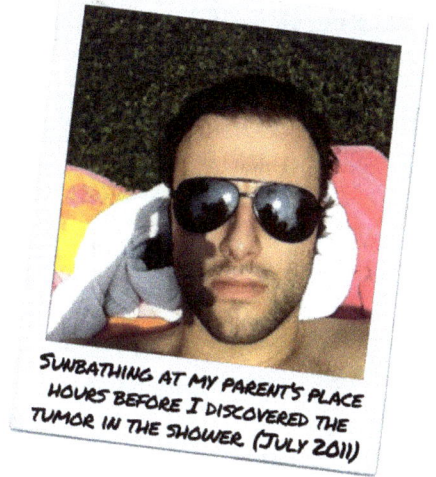

SUNBATHING AT MY PARENT'S PLACE HOURS BEFORE I DISCOVERED THE TUMOR IN THE SHOWER (JULY 2011)

who've watched someone go through treatment can elaborate on those elements a little bit more, but there's so much more to being hairless and depleted than that. There's so much more to being a slave to a hospital, treatments, and a medical schedule that isn't touched upon or conveyed by the physical ailments that are the outward signs of being a cancer patient. I'm going to convey those to you. I'm going to take what you already know, the basics, and put them under a microscope for your understanding. I'm going to talk about the things that cancer patients don't want you to know about; the reasons they wear hats, and wigs, and sparkly outfits, or whatever, and pretend they're okay while you're around.

After I do that, I'm going to talk to you about what you definitely don't know or haven't considered. Once the tight hand of hospitals, doctors, and treatments loosens up a little, or let go entirely, you start to realize that that hand was an actual support system, a backbone, a structure. In a sick way, you need it. Once it's gone you sort of fall apart into a blob of uncertainty, fawning for an appointment, almost anticipating something to go horribly wrong so you have something stark and clear to do amongst the question marks. The process of letting that need go is a hurdle in and of itself, and then your life after treatment begins, but it's almost as hard as treatment itself.

In short, one starts out as a whole person, the person you are, or were, then you're ripped away from that life, hooked up to machines and tubes for days and months at a time, and forced into this codependent professional patient lifestyle. Once you're given the 'all clear' and released, you're heartlessly sent back out into the world; set free, and the real work, the real repair, and recovery begins with no clear start point or guideline of what to do. Then the questions begin.

Who am I?

Why do I feel 'X'?

Why am I such a mental mind field?

What am I going to do?

How do I find joy in things I used to like again?

By the time I've submitted this book for publication I'll have been cancer free for five years. Sometimes I forget it even happened at all until some weird sense memory triggers me back into those box-like hospital rooms. Then I remember. It's amazing to me when I consider all the complications there were, and the depth of the dark hole of terrible I'd dug and hurled myself into during my mere ten months of treatment and recovery. But I'm one of the lucky ones that gets to stand and say, "I'm Still Here."

Everyone has a thing that saves them; pulls them out of the hole they've fallen into. Mine is Musical Theatre. It's saved me time and time again. The first time I saw a Broadway show I was 14 years old. By then I was already well-versed in the musical theater idiom, having grown up drinking in the cast albums of Joseph and The Amazing Technicolor Dream Coat, The Secret Garden, Godspell, My Fair Lady; all pushed upon my sisters and I by my aunt. We knew every song on the cast albums we'd collected, as well as the dialogue between scenes. These shows became our past time, acting out the songs and scenes in the living room with the windows open and the back door ajar in our open concept living room, living in the cross breeze.

The year grandma got us the VHS of Mary Poppins, and a bootleg of The Slipper and the Rose, we watched them day in and day out, on repeat, over and over again. When you're from rural Pennsylvania in a town of five thousand people, there isn't really much else to do. So, I suppose it was no surprise to my parents when I ran away from home three days after high school graduation to move to New York City and pursue my pipe dream: a career in Musical Theater - the two most glorious words in the English language. Musical Theatre saved me from Central Pennsylvania.

Now, this isn't to say that musicals can save everyone, though I truly believe that they can. I believe musicals would be the springboard for world peace, but I guess they're not for everybody, so that's another story, never mind, anyway. Support groups that I was encouraged to attend throughout the course of cancer were not for me, and certainly have benefited thousands, so I get it. A line of forty people tap-dancing in perfect unison to a twenty-four-piece orchestra isn't thrilling for some people... but I don't want to know them.

For that reason, I've always wanted to write a book about my experiences because I felt as if something needed to be said for the aftermath compared to the process of cancer. Clarity of that notion was given to me around January of 2016. I met a guy online, very handsome. We'd been chatting for a brief period of time before I gave him my address.

"I'll be about 30 minutes; I'm on East 68th Street and 1st Avenue."

Wait. East 68th Street and 1st Avenue is Sloan Kettering; what was he doing there? My eyebrow crept up my forehead. I wondered, but I brushed it off until after he was covered in my sweat and lying in my snuggle nook.

"So... Sloan Kettering?"

He shot straight up and looked at me as though I'd just slapped his mother.

"What? How did you know?"

Well.

"68th and 1st."

I sat up next to him and showed him the scar on the right side of my chest from my chemo port, surprised he hadn't already noticed it. Suddenly he was putting his pants back on.

"Wait, wait, wait a minute; are you ok?"

He responded that he was not ok and continued to get dressed. I walked over to him and stopped him with a hug, assuring him that he could talk about it, if he wanted to. I asked how far along in treatment he was.

"I'm done. I was cleared of Cancer three months ago."

He'd had testicular cancer. Luckily, they'd caught it early and begun treatment immediately, which made his process of treatment slightly easier, but he still lost his hair, he still lost his wits, and he still lost part of who he was. He began talking about his experience and how since newly becoming a free man, he was struggling to even get out of bed in the morning.

"Yeah. That's a thing. That's definitely normal; I went through the exact same thing."

He seemed shocked, as if he couldn't believe he wasn't crazy. We began to compare notes; foods we used to like, friends we used to like, the selves we used to like, and eventually had a full-on therapy session about our newfound perceived shortcomings. Three hours of discussion and comparison later, the nagging feeling I had about writing a book had turned into a massive open window. Like an orange construction sign flashing on the side of the road, clear as day, I saw that this was it.

Immediately I began to reach out to others I knew who had recently kicked "The Big C." One of the first gay men I knew from back home in Central Pennsylvania had just been cleared for stage four testicular cancer. A girl I knew through a childhood friend, also in Pennsylvania, had contracted a rare form of Hodgkin's. I called and visited them to talk about their experiences post-cancer, weighing them against my own misadventures. All of it was starting to come together; I had a solid foundation for a book to discuss the story arc of being a full-out cancer survivor.

I hope that through these anecdotal shenanigans you, as a cancer patient or cancer patient adjacent, will be helped; made to feel like you're not alone and can laugh at me, and in turn on some level, laugh at yourself. I hope that you, as a non-cancer patient, friend, stranger, book addict, or whoever you may be, can learn, laugh, and appreciate all I have to say.

Now. Let's start from the very beginning; a very good place to start.

I.I Where Am I Now?

How did I fucking get here? Three weeks before Christmas 2011, and the Revlon Medium Dark from performing in Hairspray in Reno, Nevada had barely washed completely off my face. Shadows of mic-tape still clung to the nape of my neck, and here I was, facing long-term hospitalization, contemplating my mortality, and Cancer.

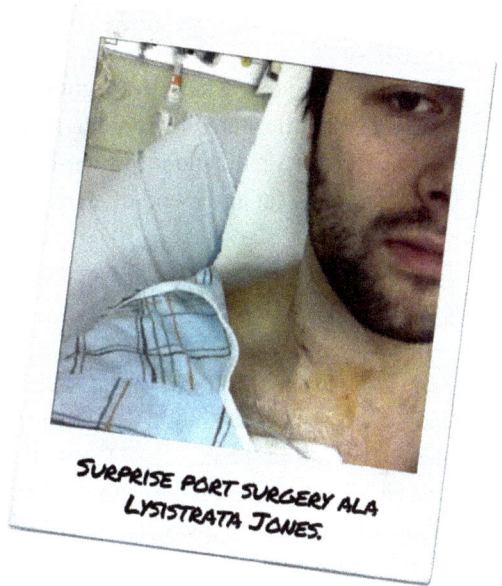

SURPRISE PORT SURGERY ALA LYSISTRATA JONES.

"Edward Miskie?"

Shit, it was happening. The stack of forms I'd filled out, signed, and handed to Myrrhine the receptionist must have cleared. Damn it! Mother stood up first and grabbed the handles of my bag. I wasn't having it. I shirked, standing, and pulled my bag away from her. I wanted to do it myself. Any form of control that I could have at this precise moment was crucial to not completely collapsing, mentally or physically. I adjusted the blue and orange hand-cuff GPS Myrrhine had strapped onto my wrist and walked in the direction of the nurse who'd just called my name.

Nurse Lampito led me behind two gray double doors into an area of the hospital that looked as if it didn't belong adjacent to the waiting area. Cream-colored walls, floors, ceilings, florescent lights, a feeling of sterilely and a constant buzzing of business. It was more hospital-like, I guess. No one was smiling. Everyone ran around the halls as if everything was an emergency. We reached a row of wooden lockers. Nurse Lampito opened one of them, pulling out two clear, green plastic bags. She wrote a room number on each.

"Put all of your things in here and we'll take them to your room. They'll be there when you wake up."

WAKE UP? Why was I going to sleep? Immediately I became defensive, buttoned up; like a cornered cat, I protested.

"Oh, I don't mind carrying these. They're not that heavy."

She assured me that where I was going, I wouldn't need them, and I could have them later. Panic. I hesitated to nod, but politely did. Where was I going? She led Mother and I down a hall, and into a ten-by-ten exam room where a stack of single-ply fabric garments sat at the end of an exam table.

"Please change into those and place your clothes in the bags. I'll wait outside. Let me know when you're ready."

Ready? Ready for what? How was I so unprepared? Was this my fault? Did I not read all the pamphlets they'd sent home with me the week before? Mother volunteered to wait in the hall until I was changed. She was being a fortress, a rock, and I was just trying to keep it together. I blankly nodded in her direction as she walked out of the room and slowly clicked the blue door shut behind her. Taking a slow look around the menacingly florescent-lit room, turning myself in a circle around nothing, I wondered where am I now?

Everything seemed to have escalated so quickly. Two weeks ago, I was step-touching for my life on stage on the other side of the country. Today, I was in a hospital placing all the things I'd packed into baby-shit green trash bags.

I placed my own bag on a chair at the opposite side of the room and draped my coat over top of it. I sat myself down next to the gowns on the exam table; two shoes, and two socks hit the floor. I unfastened my pants. I peeled off my jeans. I slid out of my shirt. I looked through the armholes of the knee-length straitjacket, the gown, a sobering reality of my location. As far as I was concerned, putting on this gown was the end, and my defenses gave up: I completely caved. I stood in my underwear in the center of the room, half in the gown muffling the guttural yelping that was coming out of me with one of the other gowns I'd picked up off the table. Tears poured down my face like the margaritas I used to enjoy at brunch with friends. I scream-belted into the gowns like I was auditioning. I stumbled over to the table and sat, heaving in and out, barking vowels I never knew existed. I tried to push it down, I tried to keep it private and to myself, but Mother heard, or knew that something was horribly wrong. She came in the room to find me sitting on the table, suffocating the screams I was trying to get away with. My face felt hot, and red, and wet. She sat next to me and put her arm around my seizing shoulders.

"It's okay."

The most inarticulate words, coated in saliva and tears came out of my mouth. I wiped my lower lip with the sleeve of the gown, and made pathetic, failed attempts at quietly letting it out.

Nurse Lampito opened the door to check on the status of my being ready to go wherever the hell she was taking me.

"GET OUT!"

I didn't want her there at all. I just wanted to be with Mother and ignore the ugly tiled floors, the scratchy gown, the florescent lights, and the impending prospects of the next ten minutes, whatever they could be. Everything I had worked for, everything I had pushed myself to become seemed to evaporate little by little the longer I sat in this room. It seemed as if the second I walked out that door I was giving up, throwing in the towel, saying to life 'hey it's okay, I quit' without having any say in it whatsoever, a resignation.

The anguish turned the clock hands quickly. Somewhere in the locked stare I had initiated with the floor, while leaning against Mother's shoulder, letting my fear, pain, uncertainty out, I calmed myself down enough to put on the rest of the robe. The blue door cracked open again, and a pair of glasses peered in.

"May I come in now?"

Through a final choking on my own saliva, I apologized and cleared her for entry. Mother kept her arm around me. Nurse Lampito stood in a wide stance, just inside the door, hugging her clipboard, explaining that I was going to have a port 'installed', like I was some sort of software program that needed an update. This required a minor surgery placing a plastic hub and tube into my chest, just stage right of center, that would run into a major vein in my chest and feed the rest of my body the chemo that was about to come.

"Are you ready?"

My eyes shot flames at her body, scorching her into burnt toast. Is anyone ever ready for this type of thing? What the fuck kind of question was that? She turned and walked out of the room, her grey and neon-yellow sneakers squeaking on the floor, step-by-step, as she made her way into the hall. Mother kept the barf-green plastic bags, filled with all the things I deemed necessary for a ten-day hospital stay.

Sweatpants.

Change of underwear.

Toothbrush.

Blanket.

Teddy bear.

I was led off to war, unsure of what was going to happen, not understanding what was going on around me. You could almost hear the snap of the snare drum slice through the silence as the squad of nurses trailed behind me, guiding me down the hall to the front lines. In a gown that most of my ass was hanging out the back of, making attempts at climbing up onto a gurney, like I was a handicapped stripper, I was headed into surgery; into battle; seemingly one of many.

The legion of nurses wheeled me down hallways, through double doors, creating a light breeze that blew through the wisps of hair around my face as I watched the lights whiz by overhead. Breaks brought the bed to a halt in the middle of a bright, white room, as an entire squad of white coats danced around, performing, what I could only assume, were various preparatory tasks to put me under the knife. Nurse Lampito helped me out of the bed and onto the operating table that was covered in white sheets and a big pillow. A massive silver circle filled with hundreds of evenly spaced little light bulbs levitated and took a slow flight over to where I was, until it was staring at me from just under my chin.

Two new nurses appeared, Robin and Cleonice. They stood at my sides, glaring at me from behind their facemasks and clear plastic space-goggles. Nurse Robin pulled a series of sheets and blankets up to the middle of my chest. Nurse Cleonice pulled the front of my gown open to expose my chest. She shot a look at the other nurse:

"We're going to have to shave all that."

The flippancy and disdain of her comment seemed so out of place for an operating room that I seized up in laughter. It felt good to laugh. All the anxiety of everything escaped me for a moment while I had a long, loud, gut laugh at the nurse's displeasure of having to shave my chest. During my cackling fit, she left for an electric clipper and disposable razor.

The buzz and hum of the clipper was weirdly calming as it glided across my chest, tossing hair into my mouth and eyes as she hacked her way through the jungle. Her lips pursed, her eyes squinted through the plastic goggles she wore, and eventually she struck rock bottom, dry shaving the remains with two razors.

Nurse Cleonice's sigh of relief cleared the fragments of hair still peppering my chest. She backed away from the table, as Nurse Robin brought over the infamous tank of gas that puts you very, very under. She dusted off the chest hair with a boars-hair brush and placed the big plastic mouthpiece on my face, dead center, asking only that I keep breathing.

Swirls of light began to slowly flicker on and off from the giant metal wheel at the foot of the bed. A swell of trumpets faded in from the distance. I could have sworn a marching band drum line, slapping their cadences around in perfect synchronicity with my heartbeat, joined the nurses. With energy and pizzazz, a cheering squad in orange, white, and blue came skip-running in from the side door of the surgical room at the sound of a high-pitched whistle.

Choreography was abounding, and it suddenly hit me what I was seeing: Lysistrata Jones, The Broadway Musical. The bright backlights continued to dance to the beat of the band. Patti Murin, Jason Tam, and I were synced up in an elaborate cheering routine. He threw her, she threw him, I threw them both, and we got into a standing pyramid with the unlikely occurrence that I was being held up by the two of them. Streamers exploded from behind the footlights at the front of the stage, confetti rained from the catwalk above, and the band played on.

"He's awake."

Awake? No, I'm in a Broadway show with Patti Murin!

"Wheel him to the holding area."

Holding area? No, this isn't an audition; I'm in Lysistrata Jones on Broadway!

"Give it up, give it up."

The lights danced around more and more. Jason and Patti became blurry and lost in the confetti and streamers. I turned to look for the audience and their wall of applause, but the drum line faded, and I realized my eyes were closed. I cracked one of them open, little by little, to see the same lights I was just rah-rah-rah'ing in. This wasn't Broadway it was a hospital.

Not two days ago, I was working at the Walter Kerr theatre, selling T-shirts, magnets, and cast recordings for Lysistrata: my part time survival. My surgery, and the gas, and the lights had sent me on an ill escape into the joy and energy of my, then favorite show to work at. Lysistrata and Patti Murin all faded away, sending me back to my new reality.

Groggy and propped upright in a holding area, I sat tucked into my gurney trying to focus on anything. My vision was still a little foggy, and my arms were uncomfortably tucked into the bed at my sides.

"Eddie?"

A familiar family nickname rang in my ear, and I knew I wasn't alone in this crowded room of gurneys. Mother stood at the right side of my bed with her hand on the guardrail. She was looking at me, half smiling, making sure that I was coming to.

"Are you ok? Do you need anything?"

Still unable to articulate full words, my tongue sitting in my mouth like a soggy piece of bread, I pushed myself farther up in the bed with my right arm. A sharp shooting pain slapped me across the side of my chest. Looking down I saw a white pad of gauze taped onto my body with plastic tubes coming out from underneath it. Gently pressing on it to feel what had just been placed into my body, I could only make out a small, hard, round piece of equipment under my stitched up and tender, now poorly shaven, skin. I checked on my tumor. Still there!

My arm slumped down and I turned my glazed-over eyes up and looked at Mother who was still waiting for an answer.

"I want a burger."

1.2 The Jellicle Ball

I nearly ran out of Dr. Deuteronomy's office like a gun went off, calling, frantically trying to get a hold of Mother as I turned the sun-drenched corner of East 88th Street and Park Avenue. Over a short stint at home in Central Pennsylvania with my parents after closing Hairspray in southwestern Ohio with my best friend, Grizabella, I discovered a small mass under my arm. Like a textbook, like every other story you have ever heard, as if I suddenly stepped into a Lifetime Original Movie, like I was Valerie Burtanelli, I felt an interruption in soap strokes in the shower. A disturbance in the body I'd been showering the exact same way since I was 5 years old stopped me dead. Something new, something that wasn't there yesterday, something that pulled me so far out of my showery tropical paradise that it felt as if I was standing naked and wet in the middle of Park Avenue.

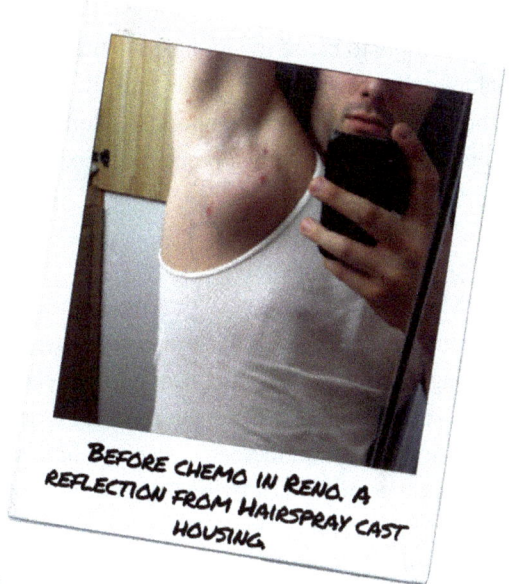

BEFORE CHEMO IN RENO. A REFLECTION FROM HAIRSPRAY CAST HOUSING

But now I was in the middle of Park Avenue, and the lump under my arm was nearly one-and-a-half times the size of the almond I'd discovered just the week before. Panicked, I ducked out of rehearsals for Hairspray and scheduled an emergency, last minute appointment with my general practitioner.

Mother finally answered the phone as I made my way through the East 70's. Doing the best I could to hold it together saying the only word I didn't want to say, I told her the news.

"What do you mean you have to go for a CT scan? Did he say what it was?"

Dr. Deuteronomy was stumped. He had no idea what this now olive sized pit could be, and after finagling a few things around with my insurance, prescribed me a visit at another doctor's office thirty blocks down.

"It could be Hodgkin's."

For the first time in its existence, Park Avenue saw sober, un-medicated tears. My attempts to blend in amongst the buttoned-up WASPs on the Avenue, the quiet unhappy housewives, the strong and silent husbands, failed. Words and partial sentences garbled over the phone to Mother through my tears and were mushed together only conveying a premature diagnosis.

"HODGKIN'S?"

My energy was exerted, putting one foot in front of the other, nearly tripping over my boat shoes as I made my way down the tree lined Avenue. The backpack I was lugging felt heavier and heavier with each block, though it only contained the script and score to Hairspray and a change of shirt. Could I do Hairspray with Hodgkin's? I'm sure there are hospitals in Reno, right? It's Reno, so one never knows, especially considering the last few places I'd landed for performances.

I turned on East 56th Street, hanging up the phone with Mother, checking on the size of the lump. Was it still there? Navigating to the address Dr. Deuteronomy had given me, I hoped this would be an in and out situation. It was 10AM and I began to clench at the hope I'd make it to the 11:30AM meeting I had with Pat McCorkle; a major casting director who sat on the board of a scholarship I'd won earlier in the year through the Actor's Union. Already my day wasn't going in the direction that I had hoped it would.

Jennyanydots, the receptionist, handed me a clipboard with a mountain of forms to fill out. She pointed me in the direction of a water fountain on the other side of the room: A Barium dispenser that I was to promptly drown myself in.

"Fill these out, drink four glasses of that, and then you're going to wait for forty-five minutes."

Forty-five minutes. Shit. I signed some papers. I checked the lump. Fuck, this was cutting it close. The cushions on the chairs in the waiting area became more uncomfortable with each stroke of the pen, and each tick of the second hand of the clock. I chugged the fuchsia liquid, glass after glass, in hopes that the process would somehow be expedited if I drank faster. The clipboard of forms made its way back to the reception desk, and I informed Jennyanydots that I had finished drinking, and to please get me back there as soon as possible.

"Please, I have an important meeting!"

All I could do was sit there and burrow further inside my mind. Cell reception in this bomb-shelter of an office was non-existent, so mindlessly scrolling through social media and other such apps was out of the realm of possibility. Every poster on the wall, every sign on every machine, every nametag on every scrub; I read everything to pass the time. I counted the notches on the clock a hundred times; there were still sixty of them. I checked the lump again.

"Edward Miskie."

I sprang out of my seat, grabbed my bag, and dashed in the direction of Nurse Tugger in his blue scrubs on the far side of the reception desk.

"How long will this be? I have an important meeting in thirty minutes."

He winked at me and closed the door, directing me to a small cubical shrouded only by a single blue curtain. There was a stack of cheap fabric garments on the end of the bench just behind the thin drape.

"Put those on please."

All the panic set in, I was going to be late to my meeting, I was in another waiting area. Waiting again. Waiting more. I may have Hodgkin's. I have rehearsal later. I flagged down Nurse Tugger.

"I'll see what I can do."

I found myself alone on the pavement, out in the daylight, thinking of a new life, hailing a cab! Now an hour late, I pawed at the seat of the taxi begging for traffic to move. We inched along, and all the excitement I had pent up about this meeting was now screaming inside me, rejecting the speed of traffic, rejecting the doctor's appointments as the former Ford Theatre cast a quick shadow on the side of the cab. Traffic began to pick up.

Thankful for the change of shirt I'd stashed in my bag, without a second thought, the moment the elevator doors closed, I peeled off my now soaked t-shirt and put on a button down. Please, God, no one call for the elevator between now and McCorkle's floor.

If being this late weren't mortifying enough, having someone, especially from her office, walk in on me topless and sweaty would have put the cherry on top of this day. Searching for dry parts of my t-shirt, I dabbed sweat and summer from my face and neck, allowing the air conditioning to wash over me. It seemed to be doing nothing. Just before the door opened into the office, I jammed the sweat-soaked t-shirt back into my backpack and walked inside as if nothing happened.

"I'm so sorry I'm late."

Her assistant, Gus, assured me it was fine, and that Pat was on a call, so I sat down a mere three feet away from him and waited.

"Edward Miskie?"

She came out of her office a few minutes later and motioned for me to follow her in. I sat on the opposing side of her desk, desperately trying to stop sweating, to focus, and show some personality. Be charming. Be normal. We talked about my career, my goals, and where I wanted to go, to end up; I heard the words coming out of my mouth, but who knows if they made any sense? My phone began to silently buzz and vibrate against my leg, and I knew full well that it had to be my doctor. No one else would have called me; they all thought I was at Hairspray rehearsals. Focus, Edward, do not acknowledge the phone call.

I pressed on in conversation clocking that I liked Pat McCorkle. She was attentive to what I was saying. Whatever I was saying. I don't know. I was multitasking, worrying what the voicemail from my doctor was going to say. It seemed my fate was sealed with that damned scan. If I hadn't had the scan, would this Hodgkin's thing just go away? Ignorance is bliss, as they say, right? If I didn't know what it was and just let it go, I could avoid what the outcome would be. That's how it works, right? I don't have time for Hodgkin's: I'm in rehearsals! I'm in a meeting with an important casting director today. I DO NOT HAVE TIME FOR CANCER!

"It was awesome meeting you."

Awesome? It was awesome. What kind of comment is that? I sounded like a frat boy, or some burnt out beach bum. Awesome! This meeting, which somehow lasted for both two years and four seconds, ended and I headed for the elevator, which dumped me out on Eighth Avenue. There was the voicemail notification on my phone from my doctor. Fuck. This was it. Whatever was on that voicemail was going to potentially be the scariest thing I'd ever had to face, including the large, albino homeless woman I'd navigated past the year before, who slept half naked, and un-bathed, spread-eagle, on the floor of the 3 train. I could walk a few blocks uptown to rehearsal and avoid listening to the message, or I could face it head on.

Staring at the voicemail prompt on my phone, I swayed back and forth on what to do in the middle of the sidewalk! Courage. Fuck it. I hit the play button on my voicemail screen.

"Cat Scratch Fever."

…

Cat. Scratch. Fever? Like the Ted Nugent song? You have got to be kidding me. Cat Scratch Fever is barely a real condition. It generally only exists in infants and the rare adult who's never had any exposure to felines and hasn't built up an antibody to cat germs. I grew up with cats, and not just the musical by Andrew Lloyd Webber. There were cats in the house from before I was born to present day. But, having no reason not to trust my doctor's presumed expertise, and a rehearsal to get to, thanks for the extra stress, and informing me that there was a Jellicle Ball prancing through my armpit. I picked up the antibiotic he prescribed to solve the problem on my way back to rehearsal. This seemed so far-fetched, and so ludicrous, even for me, but I had a show to do, and couldn't be concerned with doubt or second opinions.

I left for Hairspray and Reno two days later.

13 A Sweet Little Guy Named Seymour

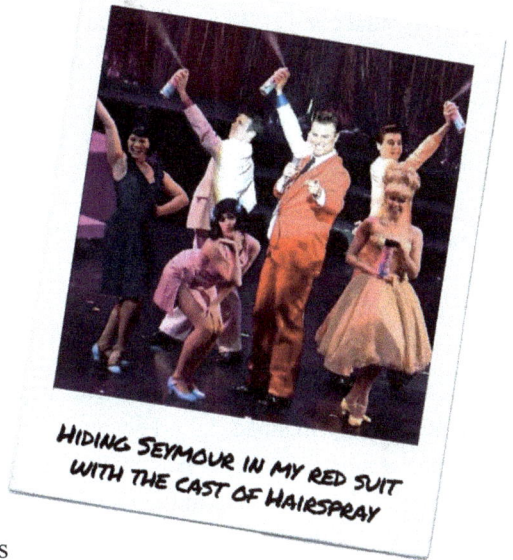

HIDING SEYMOUR IN MY RED SUIT WITH THE CAST OF HAIRSPRAY

Blowing through the double glass doors and past blackjack tables, I power walked through the casino down the back stairs by the slot machines to the men's dressing room. I felt like Velma Kelly had she just gotten back from a nude beach at Lake Tahoe instead of having murdered her sister. For the first time in the history of my career I was late and was the second number in the show.

Throwing my things beside my dressing table, I sat down in a huff and haste in front of the mirror. Oh, God my hair. Sand was embedded in my scalp. I was totally wind-blown, a mess. One way or another, in the next five minutes, I was going to tease this mop up to the heavens.

Carefully combing through my beach tangled hair, I piled and sprayed, and sprayed and piled it high atop my head, coating it with Suave Number 10. I busted out the pressed powder and frantically began to beat my face with the Revlon Medium Dark as the stage manager called 'places'. Shit! I threw on my bright red suit, taking one last scan of Corny in the mirror, and sprinted for the staircase just as that Baltimore sound cued up. Arriving upstage in the right wing, panting through the end of the opening number, anticipating my drum cadence entrance for The Nicest Kids in Town, I made it.

Blackout! The spotlights began to swirl in the pitch-black button of 'Baltimore', and the heavy drums rolled. I ran out to center stage with my back to the audience giving my hair a swirl of prop hairspray. Another actor ran on to take the spray and pass off the vintage microphone as I spun around to a spotlight and the audience; fifty people in an eight-hundred-person theatre. Reno!

"HEYYYYYYY there, teenage Baltimore..."

Ugh! Thank God, I made it. Seven weeks into the eighteen-week contract and I hadn't missed a cue yet. My heart raced through the Baltimore beat faster than normal, only having a moment to semi-calm myself over the dialogue of the underscored scenes.

"I told you not to listen to that Colored music!"

Someone in the front row roused.

"What the fuck?"

Continuing to smile, point, snap, and step-touch as the scene music played over us in the partially lit stage right, I scanned the front row where a group of six black men were seated, all with drinks in hand, one passed out. The five that were still watching the show adjusted in their seats, leering, and leaning as close to the stage as they could, blithely unaware of the subject matter or content of the show.

Shit! The next thing I was about to sing was 'Negro Day'. I was definitely going to die. They're going to jump up on this stage and kill me. Great! So, ready or not, here I go. The lyric came and went without incident, and I could breathe easy, easing back into the remainder of Nicest Kids.

"I'm Mister Corny Collins with the latest greatest..."

My left hand went up, and a sharp pulling pain shot through my left shoulder blade and the crux of my arm right where the pectoral muscle meets the shoulder. Was I just shot? Oh god, the guys in the front row, did they? Was I? I began to formulate an emergency escape plan. There was no privacy on stage to die.

Involuntarily, my body continued with the song, and my brain had a full-on panic attack. My Suave Number10 pompadour nearly became a comb over in about sixteen bars worth of music. This was not how I'd envisioned the end, but I guess dying on stage was, maybe, every actor's compromise? If I couldn't die a particular the way I wanted, I guess this was a second best?

The pulling continued through the rest of the show, but I made it to curtain call. The applause subsided, the curtain fell, and I tore through the backstage crossover, downstairs into the men's dressing room. Unbuttoning and peeling off my soaked costume, I discretely, sharing a dressing area with about 5 other people, took a quick look in the mirror at the now larger-than-a-lemon size lump under my arm, and its stretch marks. There were stretch marks on my upper left pectoral. Stretch.

Marks. Whatever this thing was doing, it was doing it quickly and with fury. It was pissed, and I couldn't figure out why.

I left the theatre ferociously Googling 'Emergency Rooms' hoping there was one within walking distance. One mile. Skid Row General Hospital. Great. I Manhattan-power-walked one generous mile in the cold desert night air to the ER. There was no one else in the waiting area; it must have been a slow night in Reno. I approached the front desk where three women sat typing away. Ronette, Chiffon, and Crystal. I asked the three of them if a doctor could see me. Chiffon chimed in first. The other two seemed weary of the day; they must have been working the split shift.

"What is this in regard to?"

Anything I could do to be vague, I danced around the question describing pain in my left shoulder. No, it was not a heart attack. Chiffon handed me a clipboard full of forms. I signed some papers. I checked the size of the lump. Yup, still lemon sized. I sat in the plastic chairs lining the windows, uncomfortable and anxious. The news on the flat screen TV on the opposite side of the waiting area reported another brush fire in the desert hills; an eerily beautiful site that rolled out like a welcome mat my first night in town. Blankly watching the news report without absorbing a shred of information, my brain was on fire, like the hills, matching the sensation in my left armpit. The fires segued into news of the annual balloon festival that was 'just around the corner' and was soon interrupted by Dr. Orin.

"Edward Miskie? Is Edward Miskie here?"

I was the only person in the room.

"Yes."

I stood up and walked in his direction through the door he'd propped open for me. I felt like I was tiptoeing behind him towards an exam room that seemed like it was another generous mile away. My face was still caked with patches of pressed powder, smeared with sweat, and my hair was still shellacked with half a can of hairspray. For anywhere else in the world, it would have been a sight to see me walk the halls of a hospital, but for an Emergency Room in Reno, Nevada, not a single nurse batted an eyelash.

"So, what brings you here tonight?"

Attempting to avoid smearing Medium Dark all over my shirt, I lifted my arm and sleeve to reveal a swollen mass that had set up camp in the crease of my armpit. The Jellicle Ball had extended its guest list to many new felines, it seemed, and the dance was expanding its partnering to the corners of my armpit. Very matter-of-factly Dr. Orin began to poke and prod at the ball, shriveling various parts of his face as it danced at the touch of his gloved hand. He examined my mysterious growth, endlessly puzzled at the ridiculous epic saga of valor and heartbreak that had taken over the stage of my left arm.

"Well. I'm stumped. I'm going to order you an ultrasound."

So, after all these years of trying I'm finally pregnant? Why the hell would I need an ultrasound? Supposing the CT scan I had in The City hadn't given any answers, what did I really have to lose? I consented. Through the empty, silent hallways of this empty, dead-zone hospital, I followed Dr. Orin into another exam room where he directed me to take off my shirt and lay down on what looked like a dentist chair.

"Aren't you going to buy me dinner first?"

Silence. Dr. Orin left, closing the door behind him. I stripped down and sat in the creepy chair engulfed in the blue glow of the dark room. Was that a black light? Good thing I washed my shorts the night before. What the hell was going on? A tall, buxom, blond, bursting out of her pink and leopard scrubs, that were maybe a size too small, slinked and stumbled towards me in her impossibly high heels. Nurse Audrey. She gently grabbed my left wrist, placing it above my head as the chair fell backwards into a reclining position. From out of her scrubs, she produced a triangular capped tube from which she squeezed cold, slimy contents onto my armpit. It looked and smelled like Astroglide. Nurse Audrey brought over a device that looked like a vibrator from Sharper Image, and dug it into my armpit, rocking it back and forth like a joystick. The screen on the table flickered on to what looked like brains moving around as she glided the vibrator over the ball.

"I have no idea what that is. Never saw anything like it."

She wiped the lube off my armpit and cleared me to get dressed again. No cigarette, no cocktail. She walked over to the desktop on the other side of the room and began clicking at the keyboard with her painted nails. Shifting my weight to my right leg, I asked if I was good to go, or if there was anything else they needed to do.

"Here."

She handed me a single sheet of white paper on the opposite end of a shoulder shrug.

"There's a list of possibilities of what that could be, but you're going to need a biopsy to determine anything for sure."

Viral Infection

Lupus

Fibro Adenoma

Mononucleosis

AIDS

Fungal Infection

Lymphoma

Breast Cancer

Allergic Reaction (medication)

Cat Scratch Fever.

Fucking seriously? Cat Scratch Fever? Again? With my list of fates in hand, I blindly walked out of the room trying to retrace my steps back to the waiting area; left, right, right, straight, left. I couldn't have rolled my eyes any harder at the notion that the snow globe under my arm was caused by a feline of any kind, Lloyd

Webber, or otherwise. Hunched over the check-in desk in the waiting room, I signed even more papers. Recognizing that none of the ailments listed on the sheet were funny, still, I was almost chuckling at the idea that this could have been anything listed; except one. Lymphoma. That scared me.

Leaving the hospital, frustrated and pissed, I walked down the block towards the actor's hotel texting Mushnik. He'd drive from Sacramento every week to entertain me and watch the show.

"Meet me at the The Two Star."

The Two Star was what we called the gay bar down the block from where the cast was staying. It was really called The Five Star, but Two Star seemed more appropriate. There may have been ten people in the whole place when I arrived. Mushnik was already perched at the middle of the bar by the beer stop with a bourbon and ginger ale waiting for me.

"Where did you go?"

I came out to him about the Jellicle Ball under my arm, and the ridiculous hospital run of the past hour. I brushed off my fears and worries and laughed at the notion that I could have a twin growing inside me.

"Well, you're obviously going to have to name it."

We laughed in agreeance taking notice that Little Shop of Horrors was showing on the television behind the bar. As if a bolt of lightning hit us both during "Total Eclipse of The Sun" our faces turned to momentary stone as we looked at each other and simultaneously yelled "SEYMOUR!"

1.4 Park & 73rd

Double booked and frantic, I ran from the A Train stop at Columbus Circle, to West 57th Street and 6th Avenue through a warm November air. Weeks of phoning Dr. Deuteronomy to report on Seymour's progress and size had finally intersected with my return to New York. The twin now growing under my arm was about the size of a grapefruit – respectively. It was finally time to have an in-person conversation with Dr. Deuteronomy about Seymour, but first, a pit-stop.

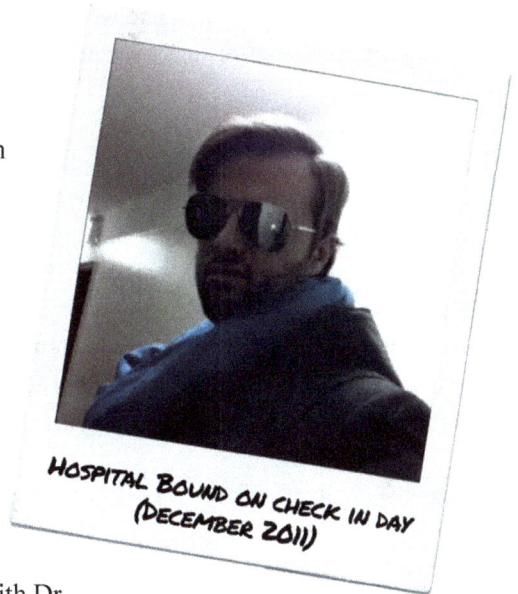

HOSPITAL BOUND ON CHECK IN DAY (DECEMBER 2011)

Genetics being what they are, I knew what the future of my scalp had in store for me. So, being an actor, terrified of never working again, as we all are, and terribly concerned with how I looked, in general, I proactively spent my time in Reno being very stingy. I'd managed to save up a down payment for a hair transplant. Dr. Zack was a Midtown Manhattan-based plastic surgeon with a specialization in hair surgery. I needed this. I needed this to stay employed as an actor; to stay twenty-five, and intact. One time an actor told me that he only went to the gym to stay employable and dateable. Was this the same thing?

Inside the elevator to Dr. Zack's office, I scanned my face and hairline in the reflective gold walls. An ex-boyfriend of mine had one of these done in the nineties, and based on that, I wanted the elevator cable to snap and throw me back down to the ground floor. I kept telling myself it was fine, this was important. I reached floor 8 with 11 as the goal, and I began to question if this was stupid, but pushed it away because I was now standing outside of Dr. Zack's office door.

Cassie, the receptionist, greeted me with good vibes and a clipboard full of questions. Sitting in the small, blue office, I wondered why the hell anyone would need to know if I had gastro-intestinal problems for an outpatient surgery on my head? I signed some papers. I checked on Seymour. Still there. I returned the clipboard to Cassie, and sat in the waiting area, staring at the before and after photos on the wall of other men and women who'd made the same decision I was about to. They were comforting. I was making the right choice. I think.

"Edward Miskie."

Dr. Zack appeared in the doorway. His hair was slicked back. He had a lot of it. I wondered if he'd had a transplant done. I followed his scalp into his office and sat down, as instructed in a chair by his desk. He began to ask me questions that I could only assume were to evaluate my psyche; was I crazy? He positioned a series of mirrors around me as he rounded the corner from psychological to procedural, taking out a brown pencil-marker from his desk. He walked over to me and placed his hand on the top of my head, pushing my hair backwards.

"Look in the mirror."

The pencil took my forehead to task; he poked and scraped dark lines and shaded in areas all over the front of my head where my high school hairline used to live. Great. This was worse than I thought. Maybe I should just purge all the money, get twice as much work done, and fuck eating for the rest of the year.

"This hair here got on a Trailways bus, and headed for the big bad apple..."

What? I was *in* the big bad apple... This is stupid. I felt stupid. I started to feel sick as I watched the dark lines grow denser. Dr. Zack's voice and his doodling's had now brought my anxiety level to a rise, and Seymour began to throb. As he moved on in his well-rehearsed sales pitch, transitioning from terrain to needles, Seymour's throb turned into a grumble.

"Needles jab holes in your head to make room for the transplanted follicles."

That angered Seymour. He began to pulse at each step Dr. Zack walked me through. When he mentioned the seven hours it took to complete the surgery, and the nurse whose sole job it was to wipe blood off my forehead as the needles penetrated, Seymour swelled and began a maddening pulse under my sweater. I abruptly stood up, interrupting Dr. Zack, using my appointment with Dr. Deuteronomy as an excuse to bolt. Seymour wanted out of that office, and for the first time in his existence, I listened to him.

Hugging the bulging folder full of expectations for hair transplant and money vomiting under my non-tumescent arm, I squeaked out a 'thank you' and 'I'll be in touch' before I backed away towards the door. This thing under my arm needed to be extinguished. I had angered Seymour. He pushed me out the door and on to my next appointment with Dr. Deuteronomy.

It was quiet. The phones behind the reception desk weren't ringing, the doorbell on the front door wasn't buzzing, and I could hear the flies in the room buzzing around the sheer white window dressings. Seymour's pulse from Dr. Zack's office had calmed a bit in the chaos of the Six Train but sitting in Dr. Deuteronomy's office kept him on a steady pulse. He hated silence. He was making a scene amongst the orchids, fashion mags, and flies.

Dr. Deuteronomy opened the door to the back, cutting through the quiet, briefly silencing Seymour's beat.

"Edward Miskie, good to see you. Welcome back!"

I followed him into one of three exam rooms, his shiny ox-blood loafers squishing the carpet beneath his feet, permeating the air with the sound of money.

"So, what's going on with this thing?"

Well... I lifted my sweater to reveal the breast growing in my left armpit. Dr. Deuteronomy scrunched up his brow like tissue paper in a gift bag and began to poke at and move Seymour around. He drew in a deep breath, and sighed ripping off his non-latex glove. His all too familiar nervous tic began to act up; he smacked his lips against his gums and stared at the wall for a moment.

"You don't feel ill? You don't feel tired or fatigued in any way?"

He asked me that twice, like he didn't believe me when I told him I felt completely normal.

"Yes, I guess you would feel normal. You've never looked better. You're the picture of health. I don't get it. Hang on."

He broke away from the wall and darted out of the exam room. His white lab coat trailed behind him, leaving me surrounded by the hum of the lights in the ceiling, and the faint throb of Seymour. I began to take up with the walls, ignoring

Seymour's increasing chattiness in the stillness of the room. If only the walls could talk through their bland beige and sparse paintings, maybe they'd have an idea of what Dr. Deuteronomy was doing. Maybe they would tell Seymour to shut up!

Dr. Deuteronomy returned with his associate Dr. Richie; a second set of eyes. They stood there, one on my left, and one on my right, my arm in the air, both with the same expression on their faces, infrequently poking Seymour. Dr. Richie backed off and exclaimed his confusion.

"You don't feel ill, or tired?"

Dr. Deuteronomy reached for the phone, exclaiming that I was the picture of health and I felt all right. Yes, I felt fine. I had just told him that five minutes ago, and now Seymour and I were both getting irritated. Hodgkin's was ruled out four months ago, before I'd left for Reno, and now I was desperately hanging on to that notion as he dialed. His conversation quietly raged under a mumble. Seymour, on the other hand, had broken into full-out "Music and the Mirror." He just wanted a chance to dance; his Jellicle Ball made known. Dr. Deuteronomy hung up the phone and handed me a note.

"Doctor Turner. Manhattan County Hospital."

Just up the Avenue, in the East 90s, was a hospital with a doctor in it that I was to go see the following day. Recent history was repeating itself. I was beginning to become very uncomfortable. He explained that because of the size and rapidness of Seymour's growth, I was going to need a needle biopsy.

"It actually really could be Hodgkin's."

That's silly. This is stupid. That was ruled out already, and you're wrong. I don't have time for Hodgkin's; I have auditions to go to, and music to learn for next season. I thrashed at Seymour as he screamed through my sweater. The lights in the room brightened as if they were on an out-of-control dimmer. Brighter, and brighter they grew, until my retinas couldn't handle them, and my eyes closed. It was quiet. The kind of quiet in which you can hear your own heartbeat, but I couldn't even hear that, not even Seymour.

When I finally opened them, I found myself shirtless on a reclined chair with my left arm raised above my head. Dr. Turner stood next to me, tall, her blond curly hair stopping just around her jaw line, her white lab coat accenting her beach-tanned skin. Around her was a clan of men and women, also in lab coats, all vying for me down the bridge of their noses.

Dr. Turner zeroed in on Seymour with a long sharp needle in her hand. He braced himself and struggled. I braced myself and held my breath.

"A-5-6-7-8!"

The sharp point of the foot-long needle hit all of its marks: down-step, up, turn from there. The first time - down-step. Then the second - pivot-step. The third - turn-around. As I watched the Jellicle Ball fall victim to a jazz dance combo, I saw what I did for love disappear under the watchful audience of doctors, as they selected my dance card as the winner in this hospital audition.

Shit.

1.5 The Barricade

From the bowels of the basement of Manhattan County Hospital, on its pale linoleum floors, behind it's stringent walls, I sat in a chair in the hall outside of the finance office. It felt as if this office was at the center of the world, and I'd traveled down passages and tunnels to reach its grimy, stark void. Something in the air of the desolate, empty corridors told me that my defenses should be up, like war was coming. Bamatabois, the militant gatekeeper of the finance office, handed me a stack of forms. They read like a surrender as I dragged a pen across the white flag-like page. I signed some papers. I checked on Seymour. Still there.

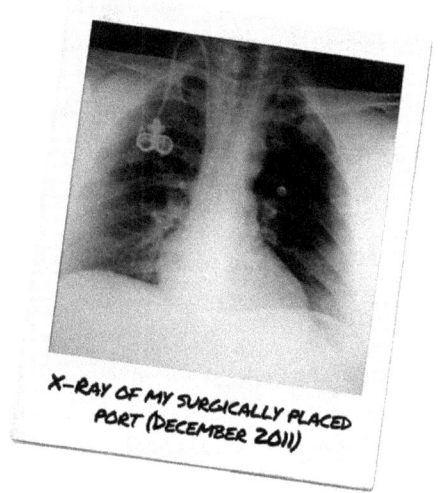

X-RAY OF MY SURGICALLY PLACED PORT (DECEMBER 2011)

"Edward Miskie."

Tucking my jacket in the crux of my arm, Bamatabois called my name and lured me to his desk. It had been over a week since my needle biopsy came back as flamboyantly positive for Non-Hodgkin's Lymphoma and a plan had been made for my embarkation into cancer land, the hospital, and unfamiliar, terrifying, territory. I was scared. I was standing very literally on the threshold of cancer, the divide between before and after. Today was only the overture to the opening number; having been prescribed a PET and MUGGA heart scan before starting chemo in a few days.

Thanks to The Obamas and the new Affordable Care Act, regulation changes granted me the fortunate ability to be placed on Mother's insurance plan as a twenty-five-year-old uninsured man, now, with a pre-existing condition. So, although I was fearful of the yet-to-come, I walked into this pit thinking that no matter what, I would not be plummeted into crippling debt from medical bills.

"That will be three thousand five hundred ninety dollars total."

Gross! I wanted to leap into a fit about the corruption in the American health care system. I wanted to go on a diatribe about how-in-the-hell the average uninsured person could possibly have any hope of living, literally living, should they be faced with a bill like that. Nearly four grand for two ten-minute scans seemed devastatingly excessive, but I took a deep breath, eased back, and just accepted the amount; the credit card of my new insurance would soften the blow.

"I see here that your insurance is pending, so you will need to pay out of pocket."

What the fuck do you mean I have to pay out of pocket? Three. Thousand. Five. Hundred. Dollars. I didn't have three grand, let alone three grand just laying around at my disposal. I was an actor for fuck's sake. I'd just gotten back from Reno making $350 a week. No one I knew had a spare three grand to throw around. And the fact that the hospital was using an upfront payment on an unsuspecting cancer patient as a hurdle to reach the other side, a side on which life-saving treatment was laying, angered me in the doorway of this windowless office.

"Pending? What do you mean pending?"

Wouldn't pending mean that at the very least I was taking the necessary steps in the right direction to make sure that the hospital got their money? Why the hell was I being asked for money? Why was money the obstacle between me living and dying; being treated and not? Seymour was exploding out of my armpit, and I was in a constant state of sharp pain down my right shoulder blade from the size of the tumor. We already knew that this cancer was rare and fast forming, so all the time the people in this office were wasting, were minutes that Seymour had to grow, and stretch out my skin, and my sweater.

"I can't pay that. Can my insurance be charged retroactively once it's been approved?"

Bamatabois scolded me. NO?! Ten minutes went by. Ten minutes wasted, spent in a progressively combative conversation with this guy peering at me over his Duane Reade glasses. Behind this desk, this barricade, under lit by a computer screen, this keeper of the keys was telling me that if I couldn't pay, I'd have to leave. Leave! I could almost feel Seymour growing, feeding off my rage. Bamatabois tried to explain as calmly as possible, using only selective notes of sneering shock that I didn't know this information already, that because my insurance was pending, because I didn't technically have insurance at that exact moment, even though he could see that I was pending on Mother's plan, I would have to take on the cost of the scans personally. If I couldn't pay, I wasn't going to be seen.

"How you do you fucking sleep at night?"

My heightened voice coaxed a man, I could only assume was a manager of the department, out of his office, rapidly appearing in the back doorway behind the barricade. He assessed both the situation and me. This Thenardier of a man looked me up, and down physically moving his head along the height of my body, examining my body language, listening to my increasingly frantic bellows of frustration. If I didn't get these scans, I couldn't start chemo, Seymour would continue to grow, and eventually Seymour would just eat me alive.

"I have to have these tests! Today. There's no time!"

My hands braced the front of the barricade between freedom and me. Thenardier, costumed in trust, and in a position of camaraderie and assistance, perched behind the barricade judging my inability to pay thirty-five hundred dollars to the hospital out right. He began to yell back at me, dismissing me, telling me that, really, if I couldn't fork over the money right then, I would have to leave the hospital.

"Well then. Great. Cancel my appointment, please tell them why, and fuck you."

Walking faster and faster up the ramped hallways to the main level, my body tensed up fighting off fear, fighting off frustration, fighting off the fucked upped-ness of the catch-22 I'd fallen victim to. What was I going to do? Was I just going to surrender and let Seymour eat me? My feet dug their heels into the floor of the main lobby conspiring through the busy, bustling paths of inhabitant's commotion to the outside. I questioned if I was to accept this as a death sentence as I'd accepted the price of the scans; to retreat to my apartment and just lay in my bed until Seymour had won his raging Jellicle Ball in my armpit.

I held my breath to stifle and push down my hidden hysterics. I slid my finger around the screen of my phone searching for Mother's number. She didn't answer her cell. The bitter seed ripping through my blood stream propelled me to retreat to the innards of Central Park, to hide and try Mother's work number.

"May I please speak with Mrs. Miskie?"

Covered in a fine mist from the damp afternoon I sat on a green park bench, just below the Conservancy Gardens, on hold with the medical facility Mother was in charge of. The classic rock playing in my ear as I sat there anticipating my mother's voice was like nails on a chalkboard grating against my current state making me more and more irritable. After a full verse and chorus of irony of "Heat of The Moment," the line finally picked up, and the home of Mother's voice cradled my inhibitions to let it all go.

I hunched over, shielding one side of my face with my hand, and the other side with my phone, attempting to hide my shame from view of the few passers-by on the path of the park. I told Mother everything. The more I spoke to her and explained the circumstances, the more Seymour pulsed and throbbed. I pressed my left arm down against my rib cage to try and stifle his rage, but he was too big and too firm to disappear into the cavity of my underarm.

"I'll fax them a credit card number."

The very sentiment made my entire body, inside and out, slump into the park bench. My good fortune that my parents were willing, and in a position to be able to rescue me in their catcher's mitt once again left my senses overwhelmed sitting in the mist in the park. The damp afternoon began to thicken out of my eyes as I sat there receiving instructions from Mother.

"Go back inside and ask them for their fax number. Call me back."

I felt awful. I felt truly disgusting about the whole situation. My own mother was going to put over three thousand dollars on a personal credit card because a multi-billion-dollar hospital in the biggest city in the world wouldn't take me for an appointment before I shelled out cash. The logistics of the situation made me so sick, so nauseated my head spun around the amount of wrong it was for that to even be a thing.

Without much of a choice, literally facing life and death for the first time, back across Fifth Avenue I went. Now a purposeful burning in my gut shot me through the entrance and fussily made it back through security as I marched into the hospital. Through the winding tunnels of the thief's lair, I trenched onwards. I stepped right into that office and placed my hands on the top of the barricade demanding justice from Bamatabois.

"What is your fax number?"

Thenardier heard my query and emerged from his lair once more, leering at me, sniffing at me, sizing me up. Sizing up my motivations for returning to his industrial den. His minion sat, still in his allegiance with this barbarian and his 'you shall not pass' bravado. Bamatabois wrote down the fax on a piece of scrap and handed it to me over the edge of the barricade.

Once again retreating from their ammunition, once again playing the informant to Mother, I passed on the information.

"Go back to the office and wait for the fax to come through."

Again, I returned to the barricade, my red and gold battle vest clanging against my body with each step towards the front line; crimson flag in hand ready to stand my ground. I rounded the final corner to the barricades center, trumpets blaring in arpeggio scales as the threshold of the heart of the war became visible. Shots fired as I entered, Thenardier standing in the back of the helm, fax in hand detailing a copy of Mother's credit card. Had I won? Was the battle over?

"I've run the card for the total amount, but we already cancelled your appointments, per your request. Would you like to reschedule?"

My mouth dropped open.

"What?!"

You at the barricade, listen to this! You absolute filth, reigning from the depths of the sewers of The Manhattan County Hospital, pick pocketing the walking dead of their trinkets, and toggles for your own gain and benefit; for the hospital's gain and benefit. After all that, I had to reschedule? I couldn't wrap my brain around anything that just happened. I had an appointment, I couldn't pay, I cancelled the appointment. Not fifteen minutes later, they ran a charge of over three thousand dollars on the credit card and cancelled the appointments.

My desire to destroy the barricade and Thenardier began to pull at the back of my eyes.

"I'm not leaving this office until the appointments that were just fucking paid for are happening and happening today; now!"

A string of excuses, and empty, smug apologies spewed from the mouths of Bamatabois and Thenardier, safe behind barricade. Thenardier sneered his faux apologetic tone, feigning customer service for the benefit of Mother's money.

"Get me Dr. Turner on the phone, right now!"

Again, I stormed away from the barricade having been told finance staff was not permitted to contact medical staff directly. I went back to the door where I called Mother, searching for cell phone reception. Dr. Turner got on the line after a long wait. My rage was spinning, my rationality out of control, and not a shred of concern for whomever she was doctoring existed anywhere in my body; my nerves were shot. Explaining what had just taken place, she grew shocked and irritated as well.

"They did WHAT?"

Yeah. They did.

"Wait five minutes and go back. I'm fixing this."

If I had to walk down that ramp and back one more time, I was going to lose it. Having just met Dr. Turner, barely knowing anything about her, this was going to set the tone for whether or not I trusted her to treat me. Rapidly punching out a text on my phone, I sent Mother a message to keep her in the loop, prompting that Dr. Turner said she was going to handle it.

"I'll let you know what happens."

Send.

Back at the helm of the barricade, I loomed in the doorway watching the back of Thenardier standing on the far end of the room heaving in and out. His weight shifted from one side to the other as the bullets of his berating pummeled his body through the phone. Smugness grew inside of me, a smugness that paralleled the overall feeling of the office not fifteen minutes ago. He hung up the phone, and turned around showing off his rosy, expressionless face. He noticed that I had seen the tail end of his pedestal. I smiled at him.

"I'll be in the hallway. You can tell radiology."

Through a marathon of attack and retreat, three thousand five hundred and ninety dollars, and rain, I had won. I sat in the hallway and watched a radiology nurse appear at the end of the hall and walk my way. I followed her. Having no frame of reference for good or bad hospitals, I began to fear that maybe this was just how things worked? This was going to be a battle, a war, but for now, it was Thenardier who dangled from the barricade he'd put in front of me, upside-down, draped in his own doing.

Edward Miskie

1.6 The Worst Pies in London

The smell of pies perfumed the unseasonably warm, early December block of West 43rd Street. Apple pies from The Little Pie Company made the single block in Midtown Manhattan a better place. Nothing in this whole world stands to ruin a day when there's apple pie involved, not even cancer. One foot in front of the other, gaining ground on the pie haven, I evaluated my new diagnosis and the list of whom I still needed to inform.

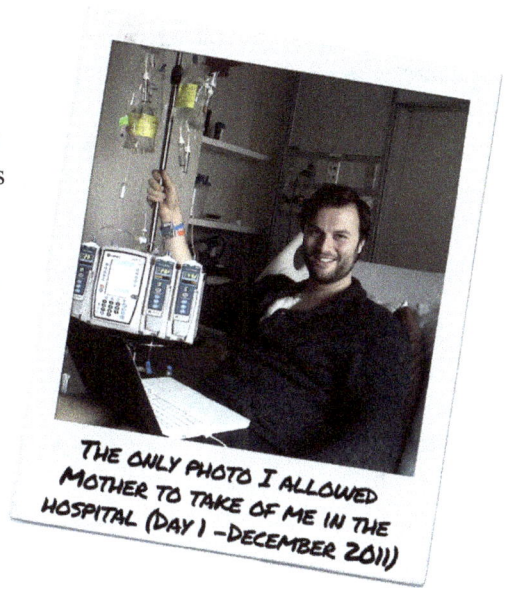

THE ONLY PHOTO I ALLOWED MOTHER TO TAKE OF ME IN THE HOSPITAL (DAY 1 –DECEMBER 2011)

"Edward Miskie!"

Caught up in my panty dropping for pie, and cancer panic, I barely noticed a familiar figure approaching, waving me down from a few yards away. Beadle and I met at an audition three years before. And by met at an audition I mean; I swiped his headshot off the monitor's table to get his full name so I could stalk him online. He was tall, and dark, with a busted nose and a large frame; prime for what I was into in those days. We dated briefly: a dinner, a tryst, and a movie were all we needed to rub the varnish off the shiny new object, resulting in our friendship. He and Anthony became my two audition buddies, turned besties very shortly after we met. We would rotate mornings signing each other up for audition open calls at 5am and bring coffee and breakfast to the one who signed us up in the first place; we were in it together. A team. They were the first friends I'd call for happy hour, the first I'd invite out for a going away party when I was leaving town for a gig, the first I'd grab for lunch when I got back from the gig. They were the closest thing I had to brothers.

Upon my return from Reno, a mere two weeks prior, Beadle and I had our traditional coffee with Anthony, but the official diagnosis of this thing under my arm had yet to be determined. We didn't know what Seymour was, but Beadle had an idea of what was going on. Once the news that it was unquestionably cancer had come through, I spent a week meeting up with friends, individually, and in small groups, to tell them about the news over coffee, dinner, or drinks. Most of them responded with such sentiments as 'well, if anyone can beat cancer, you can' and 'you so got this' and 'I'm not worried about you at all.' Well, that made one of us. The belief that I always felt I would die from something stupid and avoidable cycled around my psyche in a dizzying, concern tornado. Still, I asked them to keep the news under their hats.

"Don't tell anyone!"

In the throes of planning the rounds to break the news to the inner circle one margarita at a time, I was overwhelmed with a hideous compulsion to call, Turpin; an old ex-boyfriend I hadn't spoken to in years. I viewed calling him as a courtesy. Should I actually die, I, at the very least, wouldn't have wanted him to hear of my demise through the grapevine of social media. So, I called.

"Oh... I thought you were calling to say you wanted to get back together again."

Radio silence. You have got to be kidding me.

"...No. That's not what I was calling about. What? No! I have CANCER."

Something struck a Turpin.

"You can't just reach out to me like this. I thought you contacted me to get back together again."

The ex-exchange with Turpin left me slightly gun shy of revealing the next chapter of my life to anyone. But I would have gotten around to asking Beadle out for sips and eats to break the news, eventually, I just hadn't gotten that far yet.

With only a matter of days left until I would pack my bags and set up temporary chemo camp on the Upper East Side, I gathered that now was just as good a time as any to tell him. Approaching me at a steady pace, we eventually shared a sidewalk square. Hugs and hellos were exchanged over brief small talk before I cut to the quick. This was not exactly how I wanted to accomplish telling him, a stiff drink with the news, at the very least would have been nice, but I stood in the middle of West 43rd Street between Ninth and Tenth Avenue under the remaining December leaves and the aroma of apple pie and just blurted it out.

"So, it's Cancer. Non-Hodgkin's. Lymphoma."

His face didn't move. He shifted his weight onto his right hip, cocked his head, and gave me a sad, pity-filled smile as I worked a little too hard to fill the silence.

"So, yeah, I start chemo on Wednesday, and it's probably no big deal. I mean, I don't have time for this crap, so let's just get it done with and go, right?"

I don't even know what he said to me after that, if he said anything at all. Maybe he hugged me? Did he need a moment to collect his thoughts before he said anything? We stood there staring at each other in a pregnant silence for a second too long.

"Ok, great, well I'll see you soon then, I guess? Maybe happy hour after I'm done with round one, and before I leave for my parents for Christmas?"

Again, he cocked his head and smiled, like a Stepford wife.

"Yeah, let's do that."

He walked on, his brown Oxfords clacking on the pavement as he continued his path past me. My body and eyes followed, watching him stride away. His pace didn't change, and he never looked back. Nothing made sense. What? Just, no! What? I was starting to stew and grow angry. It was as if I had told him I liked his coat. Why did Beadle's lack of reaction, so surface, so unconcerned, happen, and why was it bothering me so much? Was I feeling sorry for myself? Was I begging for applause? Stunned, I slowly turned and refocused my attention to what really mattered: pie.

The pie was beckoning me, forcing me to drag my hesitant, disappointed feet into the shop. Second-guessing my choices in desserts, as I second-guessed my choices in friends, I scanned the glass case for an option that may dawn on me to be a better selection. I picked out the pie; the best - Sour Cream Apple Walnut with ice cream. Retreating to a small booth in the corner, I sat in the storefront window watching the leaves on the street blow by. I shoveled pie and ice cream into my face with growing intensity as I began to reevaluate. My actor brain started comparing Beadle to everyone else, everyone else who had some sort of return of shock or audible opposition to what was about to transpire. Why didn't he?

Were Beadle and I as close as I thought? Did I expect wailing and tears? Were we even really friends? I could have stopped a complete stranger on the street, given them the news, and gotten more of a reaction than I did from Beadle. Did I want a spectacle on 43rd street in my honor? Did I need a spectacle on 43rd Street to appease me? A cocked head and a crooked smile were all I got, and an apple pie.

17. Finishing the Hat

The faint smell of bleach and Purell roused my senses as flashes of the morning sun flickered through the window, bouncing off the cars that drove down Fifth Avenue. Each flashing glare punched me in the eyes in minute intervals; enough time for optimism, in their cease fire, to take root until another would come and rip my hopes of falling back to sleep out of the ground. I gave up.

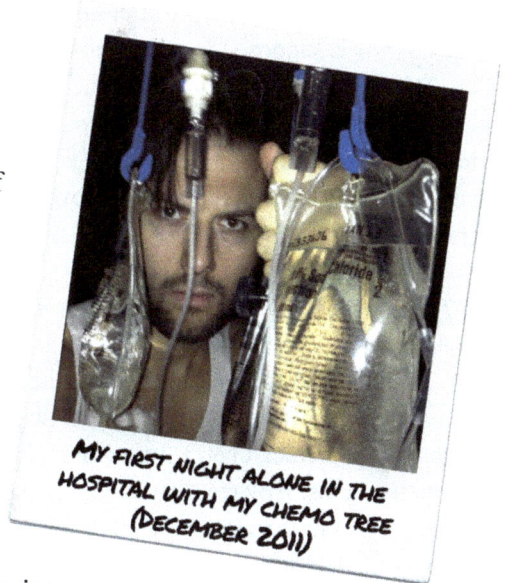

MY FIRST NIGHT ALONE IN THE HOSPITAL WITH MY CHEMO TREE (DECEMBER 2011)

Reaching to dust the crust of morning off my barely open eyes, a hard-plastic box beat me to it and hit me in the face. The GPS that had been chained onto me the day before decided to greet me, abrasively.

"Oh, right."

I was a cancer patient. As I maneuvered my way around myself, I was yanked, pinched, and pulled back to my starting position. Like a leash, the plastic tubes from the port and IV pole pulled on me, stopping me from moving anywhere. It was day two on the inside, and I hadn't yet adjusted to the tube-tether that sprung out of my chest. I was laying in an industrial nightmare of a barely-twin-size bed with big locked-in guard rails, peeing into a plastic misshapen water bottle for the nurses to collect and measure like I was in some sort of piss play doctor porn. But I survived my first night, and my first bag of chemo, so despite my poor night's sleep, I suppose I still had bullet points to be grateful for.

Slowly coming-to, realizing that last night was a memory and not a nightmare, I replayed the circus and pomp-and-circumstance of the night before.

Six nurses stood around me in the ten-by-twelve room at Manhattan County Hospital. The room contained one chair, and a bed made of packing peanuts. Mother sat in the chair at the foot of the bed taking notes of every little thing any doctor or nurse said. She used to mix chemotherapy. She was fielding errors. And

51

after we were almost sent home after my port surgery because there was no record on file that I was supposed to start chemo that day, she was writing everything down. The tall metal tree that was connected to my port was now being decorated with swollen plastic bags; chemo bags of many colors, and saline to keep me hydrated as the acid was about to be released into me. I sat there watching each nurse fasten and click the tubes shut, preventing the drip from entering my body. For now.

"The first sixty minutes are the most crucial."

According to Nurse Dot, the head of the team of nurses, the flow of chemo was to increase every few minutes. With each twitch of the hand of the clock, the floodgates would crack open a little more allowing more of the Technicolor Dream Coat into my veins. Any reactions I was going to experience, if any, were going to happen straight out the gate and I was to sit in silence and be mindful of every maddening inch of my body.

"If you feel a sudden piercing headache, chest pains, or itching, or anything out of the ordinary you have to speak up. You could experience seizures, cardio-vascular complications, or severe allergic reactions... And death!"

I signed some papers. I checked on Seymour. Still there.

Well, fuck! I could only bounce my glances between Mother and my legs under the stark white sheets of the sheet-rock hospital bed as Nurse Dot gave the official count down to release the first drops of the bright red liquid into me. Silence clamored. The deafening quiet of the room screeched to a halt every few minutes, every time Nurse Dot announced an increase of the drip from the tree of life I was tethered to. I was afraid to move thinking I'd trigger some kind of stroke or heart failure.

Each plastic clip and was adjusted in a series of pops, the mechanical chemo pump was adjusted in a series of beeps like some sort of forgotten African language that my life was dependent on. I could feel the chemo coming inside me, warm and dehydrating, promoting the thirstiest of thirsts that needed forbidden quenching; no food, no water, no nothing until the first hour had passed. As if these circumstances weren't shit enough, I additionally wasn't allowed to eat. No fate could be worse than forbidding me of food, except maybe death... from chemo... with no warning. Tick, tock?

Nurse Harriet hovered over the bed guard, opposite Nurse Dot. Her dark hair pulled and spackled tightly back, accentuating the bright red-orange lipstick she had slathered over her thin lips. Against the light blue nurses' uniform, her lips looked like a lighthouse in the middle of the staunch, beige, florescent-lit room, guiding the way to the Neulasta kit she clutched against her abdomen. It was the only thing that was going to potentially save me should one of the pinching sensations I was now grossly aware of decided to take hold of my mortality unannounced.

In the calm and void of excitement, my mind started to wander, painting a picture of chemo taking me under. The imaginary look I created on my mother's face was shattering as she stood there, flush at the end of the bed trying to keep her standard level of composure. The nurses fumbled in a molasses slow motion with the emergency kit, holding me down to punch me with the anaphylaxis pen straight in the thigh. I was lying there glazed over, tears streaming down one side of my immobile face, pulsing and convulsing lightly as the racetrack of the nurses threw medical supplies across the room to clear the way in order to beat the finish line: death.

"And, time."

The nurses shuffled out of the room one after the other as quickly as they had entered, taking all of their medical supplies with them, as if they were striking props from a set. They shut the door and left no trace of their having been there in the first place behind them. I was alone with Mother struggling as to what to say. The nerve shattering fiasco of silence left me, and presumably her, exhausted from merely sitting in a room. I hung on a fragile strand, no energy for small talk. 'I'm sorry' was all I could think to say as I fell quietly to sleep exhausted from the stress and excitement of the maiden voyage into cancer.

Eerily well rested from the night before, accepting that chemo was well past the starting line, and I was going to be hospital bound for the next nine days, I sat up in bed. Just next to me, almost touching the urine troughs, was the wheeled table on which laid my breakfast in a cream-colored cafeteria trey that had been delivered hours before I woke up: Cold, soggy mush.

"That was here when I got here."

Father sat in the only chair in the room, mere feet away from the foot of the bed, peering over his glasses, his smart phone in hand. Perfect. Eight thirty in the morning and my brain's disappointment spiral had already started to plummet. My immune system was being inundated with drugs, limiting the safety of eating normal food, and the food I was being provided was sent in on a militant schedule and concocted of salt and cardboard. So, I'm supposed to be taking care of myself and making sure I have energy to fight through treatment, and yet being fed gruel on a cycle that doesn't coincide with anything else that is supposed to be helping me heal, like sleep. Great. Morning one, in the hospital - off to a good start. But I still had all my hair?

"Could you please get me some breakfast? Anything with eggs and sausage?"

Father switched his phone screen off and stood up, looking around the room for his fishing hat and Speed Racer sunglasses. Hugging me before he left, he asked if I knew of anywhere around the area that would have breakfast nearby. I was clueless. The East Nineties were not exactly my stomping ground, nor should they be anyone else's, and so I sent him blindly into the abyss of the Upper East Side left only to Google Maps.

The heavy wooden hospital room door closed behind him. A moment alone, something I hadn't experienced in the hospital yet. What to do? I checked on Seymour. Wow! Chemo was really working. He was less than half the size he was the night before, and I hadn't thrown up yet. Maybe this wasn't going to be so bad. Maybe my friends were right. This was a cakewalk! Take that, Seymour. Be gone!

My mood had lifted, and the idea to rub a much needed one out, churned by the tension of the night before, popped up in my mind; only I found, my mood was the only thing popping up at all. Polish Italian in hand, which looked and felt sort of like a balloon that had been blown up and deflated one too many times, I questioned if I'd finally killed the damn thing. Chemo withstanding, I felt relatively fine. No aches or pains, no fatigue, nothing that would have indicated I should be rendered mostly impotent at the age of twenty-five. This? Really? After only a day?

My efforts accelerated the jiggling of the remaining flab on my chest and stomach to where I thought for a moment that my body could have levitated from the momentum. A faint burning swept up my triceps in both arms as I passed duty from left to right and back. Holding my breath from time to time thinking, perhaps somehow inflation would trigger from some odd breathing pattern, or a pinch and flick of a nipple. What was supposed to be a quickie had turned into cardio. What was supposed to be a brief escape from my unpleasant surroundings, turned from disheartening to painful as the flaccid skin folds on the side of my questionable manhood began to chafe against my hand. I've never quit anything in my entire life including football, except Boy Scouts, but laying there in a damp outline of my own body, I quit.

Unable to do anything but laugh at myself through the heartbreaking experience I'd just voluntarily put myself through, I peeled myself out of bed, and met the floor feeling weirdly optimistic that today would turn out to be better than what had just transpired. Silver linings. In the battle between chemo verses impotence as horrible things to experience for the first time, impotence was winning. No sooner had I stood up then Father returned with breakfast: One link sausage, two eggs. And toast. Insult added to injury. It's like he knew, somehow, that this sheen and glimmer that was radiating off my face was not from the toxins coursing through me. We sat together over breakfast, not discussing my morning and what occurred while he was gone.

"Nothing."

Night came as quickly as I didn't, and soon Father was on his way back to the housing the hospital pointed us in the direction of. There I was again, alone with my thoughts and my stubborn breakfast meat, with nothing to do but absorb Netflix, and dwell on a life that may not include a fully functioning genital. Partway through another episode of Man Men, I couldn't take The Hamm in a suit any longer and decided to make attempt number two at cracking the new code of release.

Folding up my laptop and placing it on the wheelie tray next to my bed, my hand made its way down to my Hamm in a suit, still chafed, but starved for attention. More jiggle, more burn, more sweat, no luck. As I lay there in the dark, clammy and frustrated, I stared at the ceiling watching the shadows caused by the beeping lights on the chemo pump sway back and forth, which was more movement than my nether region could muster at the moment. I nearly threw the wheel tray across the room as the night nurse, Nurse Blaire, a 60 something year-old African American woman exuding a grounded sense of wisdom and flippancy, barged into the room and aggressively flipped on the lights. I couldn't tell if she had smiled once in the last twenty years, but I could sense that she cared, and cared deeply.

As Nurse Blaire changed my port dressings and checked the chemo bag and tubing, I asked her how she ended up being a nurse in a cancer ward.

"How could anyone want such a depressing job?"

Through her thick accent she told me about her husband, her late husband. He had had cancer twenty years before and while he was sick, she tended to all his necessary bedside needs. He didn't live, but as a result of his death, and the guilt over not being able to save him, she took up nursing as a way to gain his forgiveness and give back. Even just to make one person more comfortable in such a dire time was enough for her.

Either the chemo was throwing my hormones completely out of whack, which, by the way, they do, or I was severely moved by this woman's tale. That may have been the most human thing I had ever heard. I didn't say a word, so I lay there, still, clammy, but considering that maybe malfunctioning junk wasn't the biggest problem one could have.

Nurse Blaire finished changing and checking what she needed to change and check and headed for the door. Before she turned the doorknob, she turned around.

"You should probably jerk off. If you don't take care of that you're going to have problems."

What? How did she know? It was so unexpected and so uncomfortable that I burst out nervous laughter.

"It's not funny. Seriously, I mean it. You're young!"

Evidently chemo completely kills your sex drive, and when I say, 'kills your sex drive', I don't mean 'hit by a car' kills your sex drive, I mean 'Holocaust' kills your sex drive. When you don't clean the pipes, the pipes get clogged. When the pipes get clogged, it's got to go somewhere. There is also an aspect of permanent damage that can occur when you don't tend to the beast. So, in an effort to avoid the indecency of a twenty-five-year-old having an accidental wet dream in a hospital bed or remaining damaged in the functionality department for the rest of my adult life, I thanked her for this valuable piece of information that no one else managed to hand over to me and decided on another attempt.

The familiar grip of my left hand took up the task and pulled, a little rougher than normal, to get the blood flow directed to the Hamm. Burning, again, shot through my triceps and my hands began to cramp as I practiced my ambidexterity. The jiggling of fury shook the entire hospital bed to the point where I figured, if I broke it, I could just ask the staff what they thinking by putting a six-foot-four, two-hundred-and-fifty-pound wall of meat in a plastic crib? Maybe I'd get a larger bed? Considering a bigger mattress, I pressed on - literally. I was pressing on it like a big sandwich I was trying to smash down into a Tupperware container. Hamm looked more like a sad soggy lunch on the go.

My head spun with the usual fantasies that got me bothered. I broke out the laptop trying to egg myself on with some XTube, but I was left feeling fat and undesirable watching the tattooed, bearded, Gods of biceps beat down each other's masculinity via spit roasts and camaraderie. My clammy fingers glided the track pad over to the X and closed out of attempt number two, returning to the beards and biceps of my imagination. Somehow, they felt less threatening.

There I was, in a hospital bed and a pair of long underwear, hooked up to a pole of poison with my hand down my pants unsuccessfully hamming it up. This must be what getting old feels like; that first time you attempt sex after you get your AARP card and are horrified to realize that this likely will not end well, if it ends at all. No amount of spit, lube, porn, or physical assistance seemed capable of fixing this. Getting it up? I would have been happy with getting it to move on its own. But somewhere between biceps, adolescent shame, and the occasional grasp of sensation accelerating my left arm, something in my brain clicked. Hamm wasn't even remotely hardened, he was barely halfway there, but a faint nudging wound up and kicked me in the juicer.

My Hamm, now in both hands being pulled at like a shaker-weight, my Polish Italian threw up without warning, all over my still furry torso. It hurt. It didn't feel good at all. If a rape victim has ever had an orgasm during their victimization, I'm pretty sure this is what that feels like: Fucking terrible.

I laid there, out of breath and sweaty, choking back the cry that was creeping up on my wretched ill success. Staring, dumbfounded, at the very, very, very large puddle of thick, chemo chunky unhappiness, I frantically looked around for a towel, a sock, a role of paper towels - yes, the whole roll - anything to get this sludge off my body because I'm sure that on some level, it could have burned a hole through something.

Edward Miskie

1.8 What Is It You Cunt Face?

The gurney turned a corner and was pushed into an elevator. Helpless and trapped under the tightly tucked-in sheets, I was prisoner to Nurse Elsa who was wheeling me down into the depths of the hospital for intravenous chemo - a spinal. Removing spinal fluid and replacing it with chemo in hopes of preventing cancer from spreading to my brain or spine

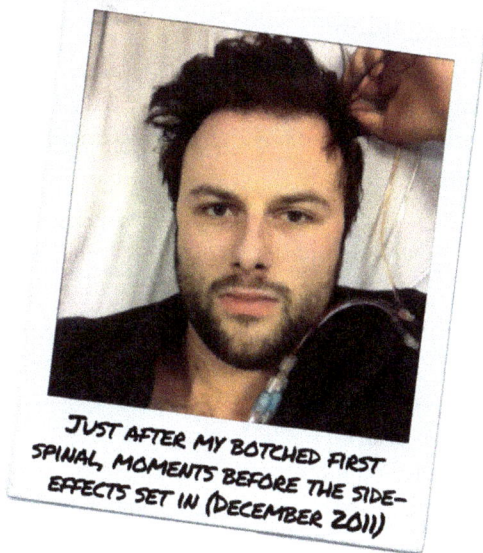

JUST AFTER MY BOTCHED FIRST SPINAL, MOMENTS BEFORE THE SIDE-EFFECTS SET IN (DECEMBER 2011)

seemed drastic, extreme. Of course, the alternative presented to me was a surgically implanted catheter placed just above my forehead, under the skin, that looked like a giant blister. I opted for the spinals.

When the elevator doors open it seemed as though we hadn't gone anywhere. Every room and every floor in this hospital looked exactly the same. I was trapped in some weird Groundhog Day loop of rooms, and floors, and chemo bags. Nurse Elsa parked my bed in a line of empty gurneys and told me to wait there, as if I was going anywhere hooked up to the bags of chemo and fluids that were strapped to the bed frame.

"Edward Miskie?"

I waved down Dr. Max who led me into a grey room. Inside there were seven doctor-hopefuls, lined up, all in white robes. They seemed entirely too young to be performing anything medical on anybody. Dr. Max motioned for assistance from Dr. Friedrich and Dr. Lisle. They approached the bed and helped me onto a long, metal table positioned under a giant machine that had screens mounted on it. As soon as I was face down, Dr. Friedrich backed away, and Dr. Lisle, that anxious, hormonal, tart grabbed the seat of my sweatpants and began to tuck a single sheet into the waistband, cooing.

"I'll take care of you!"

Great. I'm here for five more days.

Once the sheet was secure, Dr. Max led Dr. Gretle over to the table by the hand. She was the youngest of the doctors and had the simplest of tasks. As she steadied her hand, honing in on my lumbar, she stuck my lower back full of little needles, emptying small vials of Lidocaine into my body.

"This is going to pinch, first and then sting, temporarily."

And she was right, it pinched, and it burned, and I became Neve Campbell in The Craft. The room was still, with the exception of Dr. Max correcting this armed-with-needles child on where to inject them.

My grip on the table tensed as Dr. Max signaled for Dr. Brigitte, the worst of the Von Trapps, to approach. Alongside of her was a tube-like apparatus that she mounted onto the table. She began to assemble the individual pieces of the apparatus. I could almost hear Edelweiss playing in the background as pressure began to introduce itself to my lower back.

"When the bee stings!"

Fire began to shoot its way down my legs and nether regions as the tubes, or needles, or whatever she was drilling into my spine punctured my spinal cord. Of course, Dr. Brigitte couldn't access my spinal column directly. She's the worst. She had one job: to gather fluids from my spinal column to test for cancerous cells and to replace said fluid with Methotrexate; a type of chemotherapy. She couldn't even do that. She was watching the twenty-foot needle enter my skin and poke through vertebral cartilage on a screen, and still managed to scrape my spinal cord over and over again.

"Your spinal column is really narrow."

Nope. Not possible. I'm six-foot-four, and two hundred and fifty pounds. This does not a narrow spinal column make. Lightening continued to shoot through my lower body as she continued to dig past the cartilage. With a needle still in my back, she asked me to roll on my side. I was enraged while the violently prickling ends of my nerves caught ablaze with her every adjustment.

"What is it you cunt face?"

To think that I'd opted for this once every round of chemo for eight rounds. To think I was going to be at the mercy of some inept character from a Rodgers and Hammerstein musical scraping through my spine and injecting me with poison. I squeezed the carbon out of the table, reminding myself that it was either this or look like Sloth from the Goonies. Why couldn't she just get it in? I grunted at her as she dug some more. Flames, on the side of my face, down my legs, through my groin, balls, stomach, arms, abdomen, and hair follicles.

Dr. Max stood there smiling, pleased with himself, like nothing were wrong as I bore down on every inch of my body trying to stabilize it from what felt like being chucked across pavement in the nude.

"Good-bye!"

Finally, Dr. Brigitte managed to fill a tube with spinal fluid and fill my spine with drugs. Dr. Max rolled me back onto the gurney, and wheeled me through the Alps, away from the evil Von Trapp Family Doctor's, back out into the hallway among the empty line of hospital beds. Exhausted.

Dr. Max told me to lay flat on my back for two hours so the chemo could evenly slosh back and forth up my spine. So, for two hours I waited for someone to get me, asking the occasional passer-by two and three times if someone was on their way to take me back to my parents.

"I'm sure someone is on their way."

No one was around. It was eerily quiet for the act of war I'd just experienced. All I wanted was my parents.

I occupied the passing hours of no cell phone service with selfies, when the lights in the room heightened and a screeching pain made its way across my entire skull. It felt as if a tank was parked on my face. This is what the nurses had warned me about - a sudden sharp headache. Fuck. I was having a seizure, or a brain aneurysm, or a brain hemorrhage, or something where I was going to die in an overly lit basement of a dingy hospital alone on a gurney. Edelweiss started playing in the background again, but this time, what melody I could make out sounded as if it were being harped on by Florence Foster Jenkins.

I couldn't open my eyes. My head felt like it was going to split open at any moment. Blinking hurt. This spinal tap situation was worsening by the second. Light and sound were exacerbating everything. I tried to get up to find someone and couldn't; moving was even worse. Any effort I made brought a swell of weight, pressure, and pain to the forefront of my head. All I could do was lay there with my eyes squeezed shut, and focus on breathing until the elevator opened, and Nurse Elsa reappeared.

"I can't see. Dr. Brigitte fucked up the spinal. My head feels like it's going to explode, and I can't open my eyes."

Nurse Elsa didn't seem concerned. She nonchalantly wheeled me into the elevator, slamming the bed against the back wall to make sure it was fully inside before the doors closed. The ding of each floor sliced at my face as if I was a pizza being sent out for delivery. Each bright light passed above me like a strobe, through the identical hallways, and doors until I heard the familiar, welcomed, but now painful sound of my mother and father's voices.

"How did it go?"

Back in my room, Dr. Turner assessed the situation.

"The truth of the matter is, that your spinal cord, connected directly to your brain, has been tampered with, so naturally, there is going to be some sort of reaction to that."

She prescribed me Dilaudid, legal Heroin. For the first hour or so the small dose narcotic, worked, sort of. I could sit up for short periods of time and talk quietly to my parents. After it wore off, I was back to blind and incapacitated. We tried ice packs, we tried Advil, Excedrin, and any and every over-the-counter headache medication you could think of, except Tylenol: I wasn't allowed to have Tylenol because of its fever masking capabilities.

I spent the next few days flat on my back hiding behind my eyelids. My diaphragm became so disengaged, that I lost the ability to speak above a hush. I found myself to be immobile, handicapped. Dr. Turner made sure to cover her bases on that subject and let us know that there was still a small chance that this could have been a chemo reaction, which, 'there was nothing we can do about, but wait and see', except I couldn't see. The hills were not alive, and there were too many sounds, just no music.

1.9 Shining, Gleaming, Streaming, Flaxen, Waxen

An obligation to the bystanders and attendees of tonight's cocktail party coerced me into the bathroom to see what I looked like forty years too early. I didn't want to see it, honestly. The idea of not having hair was almost more terrifying, to me, than the concept of death. Since I was facing both prospects, I decided at that very moment not having hair was the worse option of the two. Death was more final and uncompromising. Not having hair seemed more like a wound, a defect that I couldn't do anything about, but could live with.

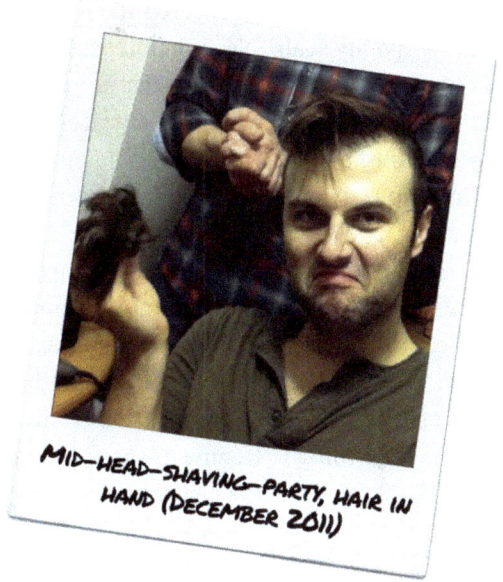

MID-HEAD-SHAVING-PARTY, HAIR IN HAND (DECEMBER 2011)

A loud humming grazed past my left ear only drowned out by the egging on of the crowd in front of me. I sat in a wooden chair in the middle of my kitchen, covered only by a sheet. Berger's tattoo sleeve guided the electric clippers around the side of my head as my friends watched one of the only things, I identified myself with, cascade to the floor around my feet. Berger had been cutting my hair for the last six years and he was the only person who I would have wanted to give me what could have been my final cut. With each stroke of the clippers, I kept telling myself that I had made it as far as I was going to with my hair still intact. With round three of chemo just around the corner, taking my own hair's life was a way to avoid a gust of wind from the A Train taking it for me.

Claude and Dionne swirled their glasses around watching in awe, smirking, knowing full well that my hair was everything to me. Hud switched on and off between the chips, and chili and commentating the event. Ronnie kvetched from across the kitchen lamenting his hair, that was retreating at the same pace as mine, though he wasn't in the midst of chemo, or a buzz cut.

"It's not fair that you look that good with and without your hair. Bastard."

The room of friends cheered and jeered at the now fauxhawk that had been buzzed into my scalp. Never before had I had such a cut; showing up for an audition for Billy Bigelow like that wouldn't go over terribly well. Watching audition and career possibilities physically fall on the floor was starting to break my spirit just a little. Thankfully, Dionne's laughter over chips and guacamole was so infectious, I couldn't fight grinning while she snapped photos and took video of the event.

Each shearing sound of the lawn mower singing across my scalp took more and more of who I was along with it. Each hair was an audition I had gone to, a song I had learned, an audience member who saw a show I was in, falling, gone, leaving, abandoning me. The cooler my head felt, the more nervous my laughter grew. I wasn't sitting near a mirror and had only my friend's reactions and commentary to rely on. According to Ronnie it was going well, but he was also two drinks in, and a terribly cheap date; one can never take anything he says too seriously beyond that.

"And, done!"

Berger pulled the clippers away from my head and examined the new frontier. For the first time since birth, my head felt cold and light, and a warm heavy feeling came over me as the spectators applauded. I threw the sheet off me, flinging what hair did land safely on it all over the wooden floor. Standing, I brushed fragments of my identity off my green knit Henley and retreated to my dressing room to examine the performance Berger just gave around my head.

I cautiously tiptoed past the threshold of the bathroom and faced the window, ignoring the mirror to my left just inside the door. I drew in a deep breath; was I ready for this? The night against the brick across the airshaft through the open window took stock of all the fears I harbored of losing my hair. Now staring at me head on, face to face, as if I was looking at myself for the first time. The very thought made me want to choke on its cliché.

"Edward Miskie!"

Sheila yelled for me from around the corner in the kitchen, whipping me around in a startled reaction, forcing me to face a reflection in the mirror of a man. What had I done? I checked on Seymour. He was bigger than he was the day before; twice as big as he was when I checked out of chemo round two a few days before.

Gasping, my heart sank into my butt. Who, and what the fuck? All of my adult life I had identified myself with an eight by ten printout of my face, and this thing looking back at me was not that. Not even close. This was not the man in my headshot, this was not the man in the audition videos, or show stills, or selfies. I could feel my compass crumbling and burning up into my eyes.

The side part I meticulously etched into my hair every day, the inches of hair that framed my face, the hues and variations of brown and bronze that the sun had colored onto each strand were ghosts to my appearance. Someone with whom I wasn't familiar was now the eight by ten, framed by the dirty bathroom mirror. He blinked when I blinked, breathed when I breathed, and looked as shocked as I felt. He reached for the top of his head rubbing his sheered, short hair back and forth, its ends tickling the palm of my hands. The harder I looked, the harder it was to look, and the more I couldn't look away.

"Edward Fucking Miskie!"

Nearly screaming from the kitchen, Sheila, once again, yelled for me, forcing me to break glances with this alter ego, this alien version of myself. Stepping back into the chatter filled kitchen, Sheila shoved a large Tupperware container at me, the top off, overflowing with little squares of chocolaty goodness. The scent filled my nostrils with familiar deliciousness; familiar deliciousness and a vague, unfamiliar-ish waft, not quite triggering childhood memories of Mother and my sisters Crissy, and Jeanie baking in the kitchen.

Pot.

No. No. No. Now I was second-guessing the request I had put into Sheila to bring brownies to the party. But I was a cancer patient. Aren't we supposed to use the ganja to feel better? What better way to pop the pot cherry than with a room full of people you love? No. No. No. I ran the list of what-ifs in my head that would inevitably land us all in prison; me being eaten by Seymour on a prison cell floor. My insides vacillated between excitement and anger that my friends brought weed into my apartment in the first place. It was well known amongst them that I had never ingested weed in any form. I was a drinker, firm in my convictions about bourbon and its benefits. Yes, I had heard every argument as to why smoking is better for you, but there was a principal linked to illegal substances that always rubbed me the wrong way.

In the hair of a second it took me to make up my mind about weed in the apartment, something inside me clicked and the no-holds-barred mode, chemo coursing through my system, knowing I was already about to embark on round three, kicked in and I decided to, simply, fuck it.

Still, as I held the clear plastic container, hesitantly reaching my hand towards the brown squares, a brief pause took hold of the room as I acknowledged what had become a personal occasion. I picked up the block of baked good and put it in my mouth.

Chocolate melted over my tongue and teeth like shampoo coming out of a bottle. Gooey, rich, weed coated sweetness grabbed at my senses and brought a small moment of familiar joy to my life with a little extra aftertaste. The Bruce Bogtrotter in me took over and I soon was shoveling brownies in my mouth one right after another.

One brownie, two brownie, three brownies.

"OH MY GOD, STOP!"

The experienced half of the room, shouted through their chuckles at my ignorance, grabbing the container of brownies away from me.

"What are you doing?"

Was I not supposed to devour these like any other desert? One brownie, ironically the size of a Mary Jane candy, I was told, was filled with enough Marinol to float a kick line. Not privy to this information, I had tripled the amount I was intended to have, but being a big person, I assumed that I could handle it, and would be totally level and fine.

"Oh! Well, whatever."

The confectionaries made their way through the kitchen, which continued to chirp over the tinkering of ice in mismatched glasses and adult libations. The pot cloud started working its way into the room, breaking through the thick of the cocktails. Each party guest taking up their share of the room, talked of theatre, improv classes, how getting an agent was agony. What wasn't talked about was cancer or chemo; a caveat I had made abundantly clear in the mass text I had sent out as an official invite.

I propped myself against the sink with a bourbon in hand, taking a moment to appreciate these people. Looking around the room noticing the people I'd surrounded myself with, beautiful both inside and out. Noticing this room of manifested luck that I had laid the foundation for, and filled my life with, over the years had made its way into my kitchen. Noticing worlds of friends colliding right before my very eyes. Noticing that Ronnie had broken open the fridge full of my chemo pregnancy food cravings, and honed in on the bucket of Kentucky Fried Chicken. I had never had it before and it's all I wanted; that and green apples. If I wasn't going to live, I wasn't going to allow death to claim me without having tried KFC.

Ronnie was seated at the kitchen table, hunched over a tea plate on which a piece of cold, leftover chicken was suffering a surgical dissection at the mercy of a butter knife and demitasse fork. Ronnie was so occupied. I shook Sheila, Dionne, and Claude to divert their attention to the world he was lost in.

"Ronnie?"

"Ronnie!"

There was no response, only the scraping of silverware against bone and plate. The room erupted in laughter at the site of someone who was so far gone from a single brownie that they had lost themselves in the prying of flesh off a chicken breast with a miniature fork. We all watched in amazement as the brownie cloud consumed Ronnie's entire world: him and the chicken.

More brownies, more cocktails, more chips and guacamole, and other such dishes that friends had brought to this head shaving, potluck, pot brownie party before we all collectively hit a wall. It was a beautiful wall, one with new happy memories, experiences, and old friends plastered all over it. As, one by one, each friend made his or her way out into the mild cold of the January night, I found myself underwhelmed with my maiden pot voyage. Is this really what all the hype was, a little buzz and airy feeling? LAME! I started to doubt my friend's coolness and persistence of my trying it as I made my way into bed.

Two minutes or sixty-two hours later, I awoke to the cool breeze from the cracked open window and the calm glow of the Christmas lights that framed it. Something that felt like someone was holding the corners of my face gently back with the tips of their finger as they blew a light cool air across my eyes made me chuckle to myself. I looked up at the ceiling unable to move anything more than my eyelids. I was here. I arrived. And I had to pee.

My semi-functioning arm flung the comforter off me; it felt like a million pounds of goose down pinning me to the mattress. One behind the other, I swung my legs over the side of the bed, still on my back, staring at the ceiling, wondering why I wasn't able to sit up. In a slow shift, I rolled my torso over to the side and pushed myself up using only my elbows, as my forearms were rendered useless. Sliding down the side of the bed until my feet touched the floor, I could feel a buzzing, tingling sensation covering my body as if I was still under my comforter, which I definitely was not. The cold wood panels of the floor shocked the soles of my feet as I pushed myself forward to stand. My knees buckled and I fell back onto the side of the bed. Pot crippled me? I tried again. Pushing myself forward to stand, I managed to stabilize myself in second position, a light plie.

Lifting my two-ton legs one in front of the other, I headed towards the door, only I wasn't actually walking, I was falling, face first, right at the door. My hands automatically braced themselves on the wall and caught me before I was a pile of sadness on the floor. Monkey barring from the wall to the door frame, to the other wall, out the bedroom door, around the right corner to the bathroom, to the doorknob, to the towel rack, to the shower curtain, I clumsily and slowly made my way over to the toilet. I made it. I was standing where I needed to be standing, and let the flow begin, but I couldn't stay standing. The James Bond in me took over, and without getting a drop on the floor, I guided myself, fell onto the toilet seat in a straddle, backwards, facing the wall, facing the back of the toilet. I slumped over and laughed at how ridiculous this must have looked to the no one around.

The hilarity of reverse seated man urination came to an end, and I pushed myself up off the commode in a sort of backwards squat, push-up, which propelled me across the bathroom in a full banana peel, cartoon-like fall. Sensing my trajectory in the dark, I grabbed for the nearest solid thing my hands could detect, the bathroom doorframe. As quickly as I latched onto the frame, I continued to fall backwards, hitting my back on the front door, my neck hitting the doorbell box, my legs giving out and sliding me down the door onto the floor. Flat on my ass between the bathroom, the bedroom, and the front door, my roommate's dog, Woof, pattered over to see what the fuck I was doing. She sniffed at me and gazed up at me with her softball size, glowing eyes.

"You saw nothing!"

I patted her head, rolled onto my stomach, and army crawled back into bed. Lying under my cement comforter, in the glow of the white Christmas lights I took mental stock of the huge container of brownies that still sat in my fridge. I decided three was too many, one was enough, but maybe less than one was a smarter decision. The next morning, even before I made my coffee, I cut each brownie block into fourths, having one before breakfast and before bed every day until they were gone. I was comfortably numb, high, for all of chemo 3, and the rest of the month of January.

Edward Miskie

1.10 Poor Jerusalem

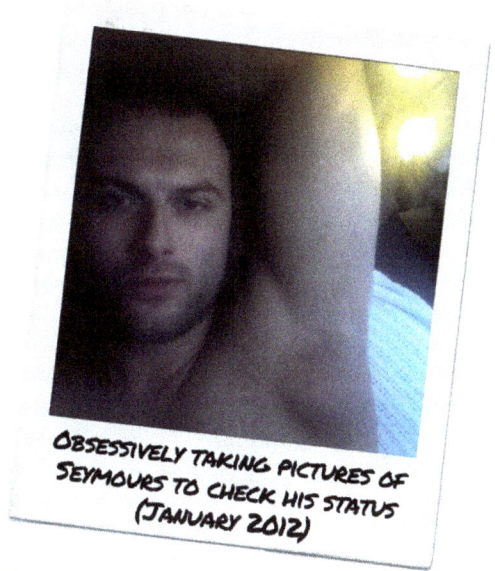

OBSESSIVELY TAKING PICTURES OF SEYMOURS TO CHECK HIS STATUS (JANUARY 2012)

Three rounds of chemo so far, each one had shrunk Seymour down. But in his refusal to be defeated that only paralleled mine, he subsequently grew back in very short periods of time; nearly immediately after I was released home. The extended stays at the hospital seemed pointless now and were wearing on me physically and mentally. The few blocks from my apartment to the bank had caused me to black out in the ATM vestibule of Chase Bank on 165th Street. I had to crawl over to the radiator against the window to come back. It was time for some answers.

Sitting in the lobby of the hospital almost felt like a glamorous experience with the cafes and full-sized trees reaching towards the cathedral-like atrium ceiling. There was a bustle hovering around the huge room in its expansiveness that felt like being in Grand Central Station. Everyone seemed so busy, and important; in a mad rush to get somewhere they were needed. I sat there sipping my coffee, unnoticed, with nowhere to be but at the cold, square, and aluminum cafe table by the indoor trees waiting for Dr. Turner; working up the nerve to ask the questions I had been dodging.

"How is this looking?"

"What is the plan and protocol for the next step?"

"Am I going to die?"

White coats floated by stethoscopes ticked against nametags, causing a cool breeze to rustle the few short, pathetic hairs left on my swollen, bald head. I leaned back in the chair, noticing a phone number I didn't recognize was making my phone kick-ball-change all over the table.

"Edward Miskie?"

It was the Artistic Director of a theatre I had wanted to work at for years. They were based close to my parent's house, and it would have meant a chance for my grandparents to come see me in a show; something they haven't been able to do since I was sixteen years old.

"What's your availability for the summer?"

My heart literally broke. I looked down at the table as he spoke of rehearsal and performance schedules. My old self began to fight his way out of the six-foot hole I'd buried him in three months before and started me on a journey of considerations. Could I do Summer Stock and chemo at the same time? It is theatre. There are wigs and make-up. Making me look like a normal human in a show would have been right on the spectrum of what theatre techs do, right? I blocked out nearly everything this Artistic Director said. My mind raced to a response through the fantasy of being able to pull this off looking, feeling, being the way, I currently was.

Anticipating a response on the other end of the line, I shoved the old me back into the ground. Like I had tasted water for the first time in ages and had it taken away again, forced to spit out what was already in my mouth, I spoke up. With as much smile and chipper disposition as I could feign in my voice I told them the truth - sort of.

"I'm sorry, guys, I'm just not available this time around."

The sensibility of the words that came out of my mouth welled up in my eyes. I had only ever turned two contracts down in my entire life, one of which was because I was in the middle of the ocean singing on a cruise ship. Suddenly, the cool breeze from the crowds in the hall stilled and I was warm. I unzipped my grey hoodie, elbows on the table and picked up my coffee to choke back the remains of my career swimming down my face.

"Aw that's too bad, but we figured you would be booked already; thought we'd reach out and ask anyway."

Yeah. Booked. That's it. I was booked all right: starring in the 163rd and Broadway hit production of Cancer, The Musical. What a fucking slap in the face.

All I needed was a reminder that I was on the brink of life or death and was nowhere near anything that made me who I remembered being. The line went quiet after a brief professional salutation and well wishing. I pushed my phone aside and slammed my face into my hands.

Dr. Turner appeared next to me. I pushed down what had just happened and put on my pragmatic hat. We sat there making small talk, buying myself time to accept and callus over the phone call, but Dr. Turner interrupted her day to discuss my prognosis, so in an effort to not waste her time, I just came out with it.

"I'm not going to make it, am I?"

Her face didn't move. There was no recognizable reaction on her face at all. She took a terribly long beat.

"I'm going to do everything in my power to make sure that doesn't happen, but we are having a harder time with this than we anticipated."

Harder time? I mean, sure, every round of chemo shrank Seymour for a time, and then he bounced right back like a basketball. He was like a pregnancy that wouldn't terminate. Coat hangers and Purell were starting to look mighty convenient.

"Can you define 'harder time'?"

She did.

"None of your chemo is doing what we want it to."

Her statement ran cold through my blood stream and bounced around the inside of my head frantically for a few seconds as I let the words sink in.

Fuck.

Seriously?

Fuck.

FuckFuckFuck.

FUUUUUCCCKKKKKKK!!!!!!!!!

"None of your chemo is working."

This could possibly be the worst thing that could ever happen to a person, to me! My entire body had been wrecked from the inside out, resembling a bloated rubber chicken, and no progress was made at all? What could we do? What could we possibly do to make this go away? Surgery? Certainly, we could have cut Seymour out and put him to rest that way, right?

"No! The underarm is hugely vascular, riddled with nerve endings. If we were to perform a surgery, there's a strong possibility that you would lose feeling in your left arm entirely."

I'm left-handed.

She proceeded to tell me that she and her team believed that if they would perform surgery and cut into the tumor that live, very active cancer cells would be released and spread throughout my entire system. As of now, and the only thing in my favor, was the tumor seemed to be contained in my axillary and hadn't spread anywhere else. Though on occasion I fantasized about taking matters into my own hands and cutting the little fucker open myself ala Nip Tuck. Mid-mental self-surgery blood bath, I came-to and rejoined the conversation.

Exploring the option of a second opinion came up; maybe I should leave and go somewhere else? Mother, Father, and I had started looking into European options. Why not look domestically first? But I was deterred from that suggestion being informed that larger facilities like the American Cancer Society and Sloan Kettering evidently were well-oiled cancer machines and the level and quality of care was lacking. The in-and-out structure that brought in and spit out patients was impersonal and placed you as a number in the eyes of those doctors. I liked my report with Dr. Turner and at her recommendation I stayed to further discuss my options. Options that, to me, seemed obvious were becoming non-options, so we sat there and discussed a plan. More chemo. Radiation. Allogenic Stem Cell Transplant. Full body radiation. See what happens.

The last thing I wanted was that Stem Cell Transplant. The description of which was 'bring you to the edge of death with the highest dose of chemo possible, and then bring you back with a Stem Cell Infusion.' Dr. Turner even brought in a patient of hers who survived her transplant and was four years out. She looked like shit; four years out.

"We also found that your spleen was smaller on your last scan. You may have had cancer on it. We saw it but didn't think much of it."

WHAT?!

Double, triple, and quadruple fuck. That means it had spread. We thought it was all in one place, but now being told it spread, I felt helpless to go anywhere else for care despite my trust in the team and Dr. Turner being chipped away by this withheld information. Uncertain if I was comforted by this level of honesty and dishonesty or not, I grabbed the opposite sides of the cafe table where we sat. Collecting my head and unearthing the floodgates hold, explaining what had happened moments before she had sat down. The phone call, the theatre, the Summer Stock season, the bad news from every direction.

"You have to let go of all of that for now."

Quintuple fuck.

She walked away as I thanked her for her time. She walked away and took my hope, my career, and whatever future I felt I had left with her. Her words echoed throughout the lobby, which suddenly seemed a little grayer. The flaws stuck out a little bit more and didn't feel so glamorous. The dings in the tables, the brown leaves on the trees in the atrium, the cracks in the marble floor.

"You have to let go of all of that for now."

Yes, I guess I did, didn't I?

How had things gotten this bad? Again, wondering how the fuck did I get here? Was I ever going to get back to the person I was before, to the profession I had? Realizing, for the time being, that the answer to that question was 'no', I slowly accepted my truth and reality as it was. I began to let go of all of that, audition by audition. I found myself starting at the beginning, letting go; first letting go of room 602 at nineteen-years-old in Chelsea Studios six years before.

I turned the corner and walked into the audition holding room that, to my surprise, was filled with about one hundred other men, all more handsome than I was, all dressed like they had just gotten out of work, all with the same contorted look on their faces. It felt moody. Who knew so many guys wanted to be on the National Tour of Jesus Christ Superstar?

I walked over to the table where the monitor, Mary, was sitting and asked to be seen.

"Write your name on the list and have a seat."

Great! I pulled the list over and grabbed a pen off the table. NUMBER 347?!?! WHAT?! But I'm early. I was so proud of myself for being early! It's only 9:47am! The audition doesn't even start until 10am! Where did all of these people come from?

Making an effort to not look shocked, I signed the paper. I checked my hair. I sat in the only empty seat between two gorgeous men, buttoned up, slicked back, and buried in their black binders.

"What number are you?"

"218"

"Well, what time did you get here?"

"7:30am"

7:30am? I wasn't even awake at the time let alone ready to audition. Who sings before 10am ever? Was this normal? My day was planned around me being done by 11am; at the very latest, noon. But noon had passed, and I was still sweating from the sweltering summer power-walk from the train, fidgeting through my music in the chair, and sitting next to only one handsome man, as the other had been called through the double doors of the audition room to say his peace. My excitement and confidence curdled stagnant into frustration. The tan metal chair I sat in decided it no longer could deal with my indignant perch and prompted me to get up and walk around.

Before leaving the room, I timidly approached the table by the doorway to gauge how close the list was to whittling itself down to me.

"189."

Jesus Christ... Superstar!

Mary re-entered from the audition room where she had just taken the last set of twenty headshots.

"You guys, to save on time, casting wants to cut you down to singing sixteen bars and not thirty-two."

What? How can one do anything in sixteen bars? My inexperience with fancy New York City audition procedures was starting to take over. I sifted through my song searching for ways to give something, anything in barely a page of music.

2pm passed. Casting had come back from lunch, and I had just come back from having a seizure of boredom in the corner of the gradually emptying prison; too anxious to leave. The natural light from the windows that lined the wall seemed to be the only friendly thing in the room, as I considered jumping out of one just for some temporary amusement. Casting had only made it halfway through the two hundreds, and my heeled boots were starting to hurt my feet. Heaving a light sigh of annoyance, I lifted my right foot onto my left knee and unzipped the side of the boot exiling it from my foot onto the floor. Doing the same to the left, I contemplated clearing the room and expediting my audition time by peeling off my dark washed jeans, and removing my tight, black, V-neck collared shirt.

"You guys, I'm so sorry but they want to cut down to eight bars so we can make sure to see as many of you as possible."

UGH! MARY! GREAT! This monitor was obviously out to get me. Paging through my sheet music, I again counted, and cut measures finding ways to still do my thing in such a sparse window of time.

4pm approached, as did the three hundred marks on the audition list.

"Edward Miskie?"

Finally! I packed my feet back into my boots, grabbed my binder and headshot, and shuffled out of the room into the hallway behind the other twenty men in the group; lining up, fixing our hair, and trying to regain some confidence. Mary collected everyone's headshots into a chronological pile. She was talking to us, but none of the words made sense; this process was entirely new to me. She took my headshot out of my hand.

"Have fun, don't suck."

That part I understood.

She disappeared behind the double doors for a few seconds, a few minutes, a few hours. Having sat in a room on a chair for seven hours listening to men who were better looking than me belt their face off better than I could, had shaken me a little bit. But now I was in line, going into the audition room; it was too late - they had my headshot.

One by one the men were knocked off the line, each taking their turn killing eight bars, I felt, they had anguished over. My unnecessarily tight jeans felt damp and inhibiting reviewing the amount of preparation I endured for this audition; none. I muddled closer to the man in front of me, and the door into the audition room. We all slid forward one notch like we were on a musical theatre conveyor belt, listening to the crisp, clear man voices soar through the heavy door and chip away at our confidence.

It was my turn. The tall, dark, and handsome drink of water in front of me came out of the room having hit notes I didn't even think were possible for men to hit and having not sweat through his red button-down dress shirt; a feat I had already failed, even wearing black. How am I supposed to follow that? Sure, I had just played the role of Simon back home at the community theatre, but I knew I didn't sound the way that guy did. Shit! I filed into the room. Why are there so many people in this room? Shouldn't it just be a casting director and an accompanist? Why are there two hundred people in here?

Closing the door and walking over to the piano, I greeted the crowd behind the table. The accompanist informed me that he had the score to Superstar on hand, so I abandoned my binder and asked him to play the end of Simon.

I stood center stage, feigning cool. I felt flooded with spotlights, and a billion set of eyes on my glistening sweaty brow. Concealing my nerves behind some guy-liner, the first few chords of my audition cut rang out from the stand-up piano. Words and notes came out of my mouth and my face dropped. The key I had in my binder had been lowered a whole step and he was playing from the original score. It was 4:30 in the afternoon and I was no longer warmed up, though I was plenty warm. My face beamed bright red as I cackled, and screamed, and cracked my way through with no power and no glory. I struggled through the song for two days and forty-five minutes. I stood in the center of the room staring at the bricks out the window behind the battalion, who were all glaring through me, silently scolding me for ruining their afternoon, and a piece of Andrew Lloyd Webber.

"Thank you."

Barely getting the words out of my mouth, I crept out of the room hoping that no one behind the table would notice the ruined Not-So-Superstar I just left behind or me. Passing the remaining men in the hallway outside of the audition room, knowing quite well that they had heard the travesty that came out of my throat, I slumped back into my chair in the quickly emptying holding room. What the hell was that? I'll never audition again. How could I, with those eight bars of humiliation on my psyche? This was really terrible, like the worst thing that could happen to a person.

Jesus Christ STUPIDstar.

Edward Miskie

Lil Baby

Twelve hundred dollars? That can buy you a lot. Twelve hundred dollars can be a lifesaver for some, a game changer for others. I remember when twelve-hundo could get you a one-bedroom apartment in the Upper West Side. I remember when it could have gotten you a brand-new laptop from Apple. It can buy you a closet full of button-down shirts, two or three suits, depending on where you go, thirteen or so pairs of shoes.

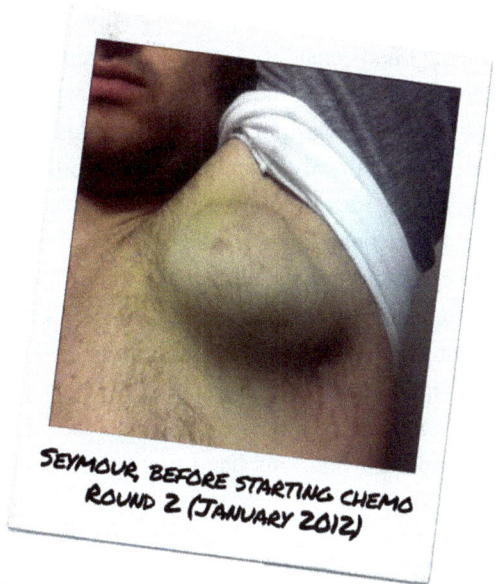

SEYMOUR, BEFORE STARTING CHEMO ROUND 2 (JANUARY 2012)

Twelve hundred dollars can also buy you a year's worth of sperm storage when the high-dose chemo you're about to have during your Stem Cell Transplant that you don't want, is going to leave you sterile, and insurance doesn't cover it because it's considered 'vanity.'

I raced through a list of everything I would have rather bought with all that money. Dr. Turner sat across from Mother and I in an exam room that looked the same as the hundreds we'd sat in before. Hearing Dr. Turner speak, but not computing what she said, she lost me at the dollar amount, and left me weighing my options against twelve hundred dollars... and sperm.

"To be clear, you will be unable to have children unless you freeze some right now."

Do I even want kids?

No.

Right?

No, I don't want kids.

Do I?

Wanting to have kids never really crossed my mind in a serious capacity. Maybe I had considered it once in a very blue moon, but for the most part, any conversation about the subject would draw such a viscerally negative reaction that I just assumed I was not meant to be a dad. The daunting fact that at my age, my parents had already been married for four years with a mortgage and a child kept playing over again in my head. I couldn't help but wonder if somehow, I had missed the boat. Did I want to be on that boat? I was a big brother to two sisters and countless friends. Was that enough? Questions of legacy and accomplishments buzzed around my head in list form, and I began to make immediate projections about my future. Suddenly I felt invisible.

Options piled up on top of each other. Dr. Turner kept talking, suggesting different paths, but now I had to decide. With the tentative transplant date creeping up on the calendar, my hand was forced to choose, and I had about fifteen minutes to do so.

Did I want to add a child to the mix?

Did I want to potentially not have a family of my own?

That's a failure, right? That's what we're told day in, and day out of our lives through the subliminal exaltation of those who are married and parents. Yes, there was always adoption, but I was proud of my family and would want the child to be my own. If they were adopted, would I hate them just a little bit for not technically being mine? Resentment?

The last thing I wanted was for the cost of a computer to be the deciding factor as to whether or not I would eventually be a hot bio-dad. Dr. Turner yammered on and my reliance on Mother grew to absorb what she was saying. I slipped away into the clouds of fantasy and began to roll camera on a life I thought I might someday want, sitting among the medical decor.

Running through Central Park, pushing a MacLaren stroller with my nearly-toddler in tow, I did my morning cardio. The leaves had already changed to burnt-orange and yellow hues, and even though the sun was shining, the air was crisp and biting. My lungs were filling up with cold every stride or two around The Reservoir. My legs burning with the blood pumping through them as I maintained a steady foot pattern and stride to the sounds of the park. Instead of pushing myself forward with the sounds of Katy Perry's comeback album, I counted the lamplights around the lake and the number of steps I could fit between each one. I hated cardio, but it was some of the only quiet time I was afforded, and I was not going to drown it out for any reason.

Dean reclined peacefully in his Ralph Lauren polo attire, bouncing to the beat of the stroller as I rounded the home stretch of my run. He was so well behaved; quiet, occasionally giggly. Parents always say that they feel blessed to have the child they have, and whereas I am sure that is true in some cases, I felt particularly grateful to have been bestowed with a content and lovely child. Never having to worry if he was going to have an outburst in the theatre should he and his dad come to see me in a show. Tantrums in various stores or public places were nearly guaranteed to never happen, though I couldn't count on that entirely seeing as Dean was only a year and a half; or as the other mothers of the Upper West would say, 'eighteen months.'

Back in our three-bedroom apartment with a wrap-around terrace, is my husband, Alan, preparing our traditional steak and eggs Sunday breakfast. He was likely already showered and dressed in his weekend anti-office attire, though his hair was definitely still perfectly parted to the side, thick with flecks of salt peering out from under the dime-size dollop of gel he combed in. Sundays are our only day together. The only day I wasn't filming an episode of my TV series, now in its third season, or at The Broadhurst Theatre co-starring in the revival of The Scarlet Pimpernel that had been running, now, for five years. Sunday is the only day Alan isn't taking meetings or clients to dinner from the investment firm that his best friend and he started from the ground up five years prior. It's our sacred day together. I always take Sundays off.

I finished my run, exiting the Central Park West side, nearly collapsing over on the handles of the three-wheeled stroller. I really fucking hate cardio. Taking a final deep breath in a stand still, I pushed the stroller forward, blaming the child.

"Come on Dean, let's go!"

We stroll home down the tree-lined, townhouse flanked street. The fallen leaves of autumn kicking up around the wheels of my over-priced, but worth-it stroller. Levain Bakery overpowered the block even as far over as Columbus Avenue, giving me a sense of what Heaven must smell like. It requires the will of a God to walk past Levain and not go in. Your nostrils fill up with the warm smell of cookies at every inhalation. Especially on a day as crisp as this one, it warms you from the inside out with their chocolaty molten perfection. My routine commutes past the bakery were rarely a struggle. I was a fortress to those cookies depending on my mood, or the day of the week, or the time of day. But my parents were coming to visit for the weekend, and I thought it would be nice to have a variety of their oatmeal, and chocolate chip walnut on hand for their stay. So, I gave in and joined the back of the endless line.

"Hey, Lizzie, it's Edward. I'm outside."

The bakery salesgirl, Lizzie, as we had come to know her over the years, took my order over the phone. With two white bags in her hand, she ran up the stairs past the fist-sized cookie hopefuls and handed me twelve million calories of utopian bliss. Bending at the waist, peering into the Maclaren at Dean, she grabbed him by his chubby wrist.

"Hi, Deany-Weeny. Hi, Deany-Weeny."

I hated when Lizzie called him that, but I let it slide; she would always slip us an extra cookie or two when we did decide to stop in. After some brief small talk, a cash tip for her help, and a hug, we bid her a good day.

Sakarian, our Ukrainian doorman, greets Dean and I with a smile and a wave of his white gloved hand propping the rod iron and glass front door open. He scurries past the stroller wheels, his long, charcoal uniform coat trailing behind him, making it to the elevator just in time to hold the door open for my son and I to squeeze through. Before the doors close, I hand one of the caloric-hate-fest cookies to him. I lift Dean out of the stroller with one arm and fold up the complicated Maclaren with the other. That was a skill that took longer than I'd care to admit to master.

I open the front door of the apartment, hating that the mud room is right next to the kitchen, but love that, on Sundays, the first thing I see when I open the door is Alan hunched over the stainless-steel counter tops plating breakfast. The eggs are always on top of the steak. He makes them perfectly. It's why I said 'yes' in the first place. The three of us sit around the wooden kitchen table made from a tree we cut down on a camping trip to The Catskills the year we got married. We commissioned it as a wedding gift from one of his friends that makes custom furniture.

After breakfast, we all pile up on the sofa, half watching the news in the morning sun, half sleeping. After several hours I initiate getting up. I hate lying around for too long, I get antsy and feel like I should be doing something. Alan rolls his eyes and smiles, his teeth so perfectly white, showing off the dreamy gap between his two front teeth. He grabs Dean, and sits up, grunting at the prospect of doing anything at all on this beautiful Sunday.

As I walk up the two stairs separating the living room from the kitchen to put a kettle of tea on, I pick up my iPhone 11GSX to two notifications. One is breaking news of the latest successes of our new President, Elizabeth Warren. She and Brian Sim charged their way into The White House as the first female and gay politician to run the country just last year. The second notification is from Father. He and Mother are at Penn Station grabbing a cab uptown to our apartment.

"Alan, they're on their way!"

Sakarian, even knowing my parents, still calls up to let me know they're coming. He knows we like a little warning when the folks are coming up, lest he forget the anniversary incident, also known as the afternoon Dean, was 'conceived.'

Mother knocks on the door, and before I even open it, I smiled. I love my parents. I love when they came to visit. I love that I was able to pass on the family name as my grandfather had hounded me about doing since I was a teenager. Opening the door to see my parents was always something I consciously clocked as the number one thing I would miss about having them visit, or going back to Pennsylvania to visit them, once age had gotten the better of them.

Hugs and hellos move into the living room with Alan and Dean, where Mother took over and picks up the little guy, smothering him with kisses. She walks him over to the windows and bounces him off her hip, repeating 'hello, hello, hello' to him while Father and Alan sit on the couch discussing Father's new album of acoustic guitar original songs.

I look around at my family: Mother and Father, my husband, my son. The only thing better than this would be Christmas with Crissy and Jeanie, and their families, all standing around the kitchen, chatting away while the kids played in the living room. It had become tradition to fly them up to The City from their respective homes once I was able to afford, force, and ambush them with plane tickets.

"So, what do you want to do?"

Huh? What?

Oh right. Back in the hospital. Facing the reality of my legacy being poisoned out of me, I suddenly saw the cinematic version of my life get torched right in front of me in the form of Dr. Turner.

"I'll give you a few minutes"

Dr. Turner left the room. What did I want to do? What I didn't want to do was be trapped in the hospital room with Mother discussing the topic of sperm. I moved past the discomfort of the subject matter and leveled with myself.

I'd never have a financier entrepreneur as a husband. I'd never own a three-bedroom condo with a wrap-around terrace, especially in the Upper West Side of Manhattan. The Scarlet Pimpernel would never run for five years, especially with me in it, and I'd never get expedited service at Levain no matter how many times I indulged myself there. I'd never do cardio outside, especially around Central Park; I fucking hate cardio. My sisters, parents, and I would rarely be in the same place for Christmas. And lastly, the son I had so quickly planned, dapper in his Ralph Lauren and Maclaren stroller, vanished.

I kept my twelve hundred dollars.

1.12 The Old Razzle Dazzle

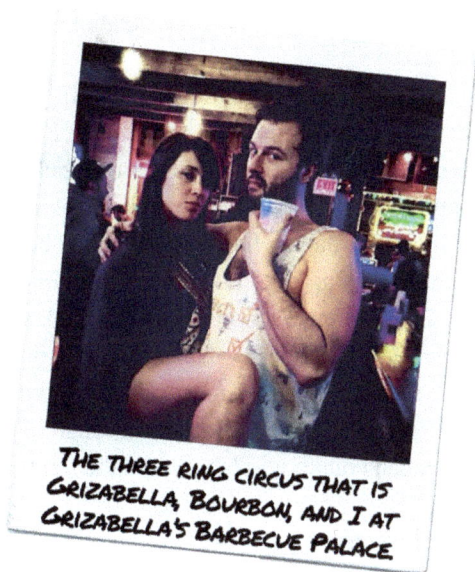

THE THREE RING CIRCUS THAT IS GRIZABELLA, BOURBON, AND I AT GRIZABELLA'S BARBECUE PALACE

Ladies and gentleman, welcome to the Upper East Side's Manhattan County Hospital. Step right up to the big top where they're hungry to entertain you, hungry to prove their worth, and willing to try anything; almost. Are you excited? Are you just dying to see what they can do? Are you just dying to sit and watch the den of doctors dazzle your senses, overwhelm you with needles, port flushes, and prophylaxis? Or, are you just dying?

Sit back in your lumpy lap of luxury hospital bed - isn't this real estate fabulous? - and allow me to introduce the star of our show, our own little Circus Freak! He's big, bigger than ever, bald, bloated, and riddled with cancer that just won't go away. You may know him as Edward Miskie, but tonight he's ours; our freak show, eager to entertain you at any cost!

Turn your attentions to Nurse Roxy in her beautiful waist length lavaliere. She's hungry to perform and willing to do just about anything for attention with her pretty, clear bags of poison. See how she hangs it with care-ish as she expertly screws the port-tubes to our Star? Well done, Roxy! Someday, you're gonna be a star, kid!

"Wait!"

I'm sorry, Mother, but you're not allowed to interrupt the show!

"Does that look like it's draining to you?"

Whoopsies! Nurse Roxy just can't do it alone! You better make your way back into the ring, kid, and let those toxins flow! Do you have any final words for our Star, Roxy?

"Good luck to ya!"

NURSE ROXY, EVERYBODY!

Next up, ladies, gentleman, Dr. Billy Flynn and the Spinal Saw Rag! Watch Mr. Mouthpiece himself, the mute Dr. Flynn in the center ring. His beautiful black scrubs covered in printed flames of fabulousness, has taken over the Von Trapp's Family Practice of shoving needles into spinal columns. Now on his sixth spinal with our Star, all as flawless as the one before, he will be performing his famous Spinal Saw Rag of intravenous chemo injections one more time, and just for you.

Let's get our Star on the slab, face down, and ready for the grand illusion to begin. See how Dr. Flynn so accurately numbs the spine, ready for the needles to poke through the skin and cartilage, all without saying a word? There's needle number one! Watch, as it bores through to the source - to the spine! Wait! Dr. Flynn can't make it in? Bring out the lightning bolts and try again!

"I can feel that!"

A hush falls over the crowd.

"Shut up, dummy!"

LADIES AND GENTLEMEN, Dr. Flynn SPEAKS!

Ignore The Circus Freak, ladies and gentleman! Under such strain and circumstances, he's not making much sense anymore. Don't mind a word he says because here comes needle number two! Watch Dr. Flynn drill into the lumbar, drilling, sawing away in search of the pipeline to our Star's brain!

Failed again! Dr. Flynn must be having an off day today! Bring out the lightning bolts!

"I can still feel that!"

Ladies and Gentlemen, clearly this is part of the show. Every circus has a sawing-in-half act. Our Star is doing just fine! See Dr. Flynn's steady hands saw further, and further into our Stars back? Severing him in half... Severing him in... Severing him.... Severing...

My friends, for some reason this isn't working. For some reason this 'rag' isn't playing out. Let's try another area of the spine and really push, and saw our way through; force it if necessary! You're going to get your money's worth, you beautiful people, I promise!

Dr. Flynn! Move up his spine, move down his spine, move inward, and harder still, inward. Push the pressure of the needle against his back. Push the sharp, metal spear farther into the cartilage. First in the second lumbar, then the third, then the fourth searching for a way to success against the calloused over scar tissue. Ignore the shooting pains of lightning coursing through the freak's body.

"STOP! JUST STOP!"

Ohh! The little freak is angry. It looks like they both reached for the needle; they both reached for the saw. Perhaps it's the nerves Dr. Flynn keeps striking? Let's hear some applause, folks, for the freak on the slab! Isn't he fabulous? But, that Dr. Flynn? This trick must be broken, friends, so we're going to discontinue this feature and give our Star a break now.

No more spinals for you! It was good while it lasted, everyone!

Let's get Nurse Roxy in here. Put her name on your lips, folks! We need her to wheel our little Star here, back to his room.

In the meantime, let's break the mood and slow things down, under the Big Top here at Manhattan County Hospital, with Nurse Hunyak and her Antibiotic Ballet.

See how she floats on the tips of her toes balancing pills off of her pinkies. Watch her spin and soutenu; watch her dance and dip! Notice the liquidity of her movements, graceful and grounded. Watch her dance in tandem with her big white pills as she presents the medication to our Star.

"Shouldn't that be in a liquid IV drip?"

MOTHER! You are not allowed to interrupt the circus. How dare you break flow of the Antibiotic Ballet. You have changed Nurse Hunyak's dance into a rage. She's thrown the pills away. Hope you didn't need those! MOTHER! You are becoming quite a nuisance to this show. I'm going to have to ask to leave the tent and leave us with our Star. But you, Edward, you may not leave yet. Your discharge papers need to be signed by Dr. Turner and she's not giving autographs today. The show will continue.

Ladies and Gentleman, let's give everyone a roaring round of applause! Fill this room with some excitement, and never mind our deterring interruptions, because here comes the headlining hero of the ring, Nurse Velma Kelly! Velma has taken Roxy's place with a new, beautiful bag of chemo, just for our Circus Freak. She's here to assist our Star in a never-before-seen escape act, an escape from a straitjacket while submerged in a vat of chemotherapy. Only when he is free will he be let go to roam the streets outside of his cage and our circus tent. Let's give him a seat in a comfy little chair, hook him up to the latest bag of Chemo, and slip him into the buckled and clasped straitjacket of death.

Inhabitants of the audience, if you get bored, or think we are going too slowly, please shout and cheer! Our Star has six hours to finish the chemo drip and struggle free.

Nurse Velma! Do you have any words for our Star?

"You're the 'cat's meow'!"

YES! Now, let's wow the crowd again! Release the drip in POP, SIX, SQUISH, GO!

Straight out the gate our little freak seems irritable, slumped over in the recliner, barely attempting to make his way out of the jacket. Poor little guy! That's just unacceptable. I know what you beautiful audience members have paid for these seats! Let's amp things up a bit, and bring some life to the party, shall we? Nurse Velma! Crank up the drip of that bag from fifteen to one hundred and fifty cubic centimeters per hour; ten times the prescribed rate. Who's ready for some showbiz homicide? Who's ready to see the fasted chemo flush to ever occur? Let me hear some applause, ladies and gents! What do you think, Sunshine? More?

"Keep looking!"

You heard the prowess of press; do as Ms. Sunshine says! Keep looking!

You're all such a magnificent audience. Your cheers and jeers must be fueling our Star's enthusiasm for showmanship. This increased speed must be motivating him to play to your needs and attempt an escape with vigor and tenacity. See how he struggles and sweats through the burn of the chemo making its presence known in his overused veins! See how he elbows and nudges the fabric of the straitjacket to give you what you want!

But wait!

Well, well, well ladies and gentleman, who do we have here? Could it be the beautiful and buxom Grizabella? Surely, she wouldn't interrupt the escape act! Surely, she wouldn't break into our circus and unravel our illusions. She should know better than that! Maybe she snuck in through the backstage door. Nurse Velma, get rid of this intruder, she's disturbing the show!

OH, MY SUNSHINE, Velma! HURRY! Grizabella has unhooked the straitjacket and has stolen the autographed discharge forms from Dr. Turner! They're escaping! They're headed for the front of the tent! They're headed for Grizabella's Barbeque Palace!

STOP THEM!

THEY'VE ESCAPED!

Ladies and Gentleman, we've lost our Star! I can only refer to Dr. Turner for instruction of how to continue the show. What should we do?

"He may go. He can have a drink, or two, as long as he doesn't go crazy."

WELL, THEN!

Patrons of the Grizabella's Barbeque Palace, pay attention as the freak show Star of Manhattan County Hospital drinks his way down the bar, and through each of these jars. Can he? Will he? Can he manage to handle The Number Seventeen - seventeen mason-jars of bourbon and ginger ale lining the wooden planks of the bar?

Watch him balance down the tightrope above the plank and suck down each and every one of these liquid fires, mixing them every so carefully with the chemo raging through his veins.

SPOTLIGHTS!

He's made it through four... He's made it through nine... He's made it through eleven... Ladies and gentleman he's made it through fifteen and he's still standing. Can he do it? Will he do it?

RAZZLE DAZZLE 'EM! He's done all seventeen! What a champion! What a feat! What a pay off! What a show, folks! You've made a fantastic audience. I hope you've enjoyed our old three-ring circus of misfired chemo, our sawing-in-half trick, our dream ballet, our escape act, and the final tightrope, drowning finale! Thank you for coming to the Manhattan County Hospital Circus. Your taxis are waiting outside.

1.13 Over the Wall

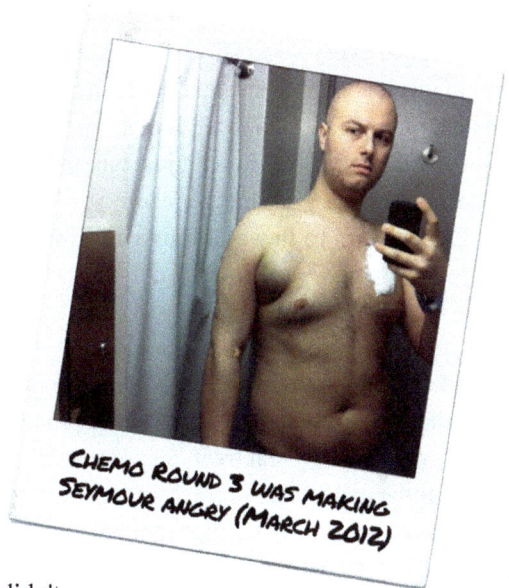

CHEMO ROUND 3 WAS MAKING SEYMOUR ANGRY (MARCH 2012)

She was inherently cool. Her pant and skirt suits changed weekly, carried around by a rainbow of strapped heels, which led me to believe her closet was likely bigger than her apartment, or she had a separate apartment that was strictly for clothes and shoes. She never wore tights. They constricted her crunchy Seattle vibe. Part of me was always surprised to see that she had shaved her legs, something that just didn't seem like she'd trouble herself with, though the badass giraffe tattoos illustrated on her calves likely appreciated the gesture. Her understated humor, her qualm-less smile shining through her unwashed, shoulder-length, mousy, brown hair made me believe that in another lifetime, maybe she and I would have been friends. But those aspirations were squelched by our doctor-patient relationship. I liked her as my therapist. I liked Dr. Aurora. She was like a hipster librarian.

Her office was just off Columbus Circle; a small studio apartment-sized haven filled with mismatched furniture and books. It felt like a home; it felt comfortable. It reminded me of my first apartment in The City with the furniture I bought at Pier 1 complimenting or clashing against the furniture I'd find on the sidewalk, tossed out by its former owner. There was something so homey and chic about it despite the temporary sentence it fulfilled on the side of the street. I sat on her over-stuffed olive sofa like a cat, perched in the direct sunlight from the adjacent window with my legs folded up sidesaddle, a coffee in hand from the Starbucks downstairs, a defense mechanism. Something I could physically distract myself with, fidgeting at the sleeve and lid.

"How do you feel?"

How do I feel? Well, I'm sitting in a therapist's office on 'the' couch. Me! Me, who avoided every suggestion of therapy or support groups since day one of this fiasco, this inconvenience, had given in to the very thing I had refused. So that was a defeat on my part, and it felt like it. Therapy was ridiculous. I didn't need therapy. I was wasting my time. I could just talk to my parents about all of this: this stuff I didn't want to talk to a stranger about.

The outward truth was a figment I avoided. The actual truth? How was I?

Well...

The fear of actually dying had become more and more of a reality as chemo and radiation pressed on. I'd started the process of making funeral arrangements for myself, which was a real treat, pleasure, and joy. I watched the entire series of Mad Men in three days. That's how I was. Cancer was kicking my ass. I hated the way I looked. I was regularly hiding from being in public and anyone who was not on my approved list of visitors at the hospital, surrounding myself only with people and things that could distract me from the everyday unpleasantries of hospitals and doctors.

Every morning I would wake up and feel like a human for about five seconds. I loved those five seconds. What auditions do I have today? What time can I make it to the gym? Coffee! Then a tingly rush would slide its way down my body like one of those water massage tables at the mall or Planet Fitness slamming me back into reality. It was crippling. All of the oxygen was sucked out of my lungs, and I'd lie there blankly starring out the window at the apartment across the airshaft. It wasn't a bad dream. I was still in the small little bedroom in The Heights lying in a bed where my head and my feet touched the opposing walls. I was still chained to insurance, prescriptions, and appointments. I was still a cancer patient.

After my five seconds of freedom had passed, I'd compulsively check on Seymour to see if he had gotten any smaller in my sleep. How much longer would I have to be living this cancer life, or living at all? I'd reach under my arm and as discerningly as I could possibly be, calculate against what I remembered Seymour feeling like the night before, the hour before, five minutes ago, weary of the tender radiated skin now turned raw, red, and black. I increasingly became more crazed and obsessed with poking at Seymour as if I was checking on a turkey in the oven for a holiday feast. Only I felt more like Anne Frank in her attic with a Nazi tumor invasion - "Are they still there?" They were still there.

"I'm great, thank you! How are you?"

Through a series of light-hearted stories of near death subliminally conveying to her that I was completely unhinged, I giggled through the relay of the last few months. Hearing the words coming out of my mouth mismatching the inflections they were paired to, it dawned on me that I was barely hanging on by a mental thread. The grueling and gravely turned circumstances of my health situation had done more of a number on me than I'd originally thought. I was in shambles, exhausting myself, pulling out all the stops to come across as totally grounded, baring down to remain steady and sturdy in Dr. Aurora's eyes. Trying desperately to keep up appearances smiling through her questions knowing full well that I looked like a cracked-out sausage with rubber bands around it stuffed into a sweater casing. I laughed through my explanations of prognosis trying to make light of what was happening to me, to find or point out any silver lining I could. I made excuses about myself, life and death and fear. Keeping it together and failing.

"Are you dating anyone? How does he feel about all of this?"

Fuck.

Well. I was dating someone...

We'd met in Ohio while I was doing Hairspray with Grizabella. I hadn't been in the Midwest for more than a few hours before I was agreeing to a threesome with a salt-and-peppered, blue eyed forty-something, and his friend Valentine, a six-foot-ten blonde with three massive legs, and a memory for film history. The threesome didn't last much past hello, quickly turning into a twosome, hosting a current of chemistry between Valentine and me.

As the show crept forward on the calendar, and Hairspray molded itself into a routine blur of beer, wings, and step-touch, ponying, Valentine and I avoided the reality that soon it would all be over. With overnights that involved ways of figuring out how to fit a six-foot-ten man and a six-foot-four man into a twin-size bed, we became comfortable, but we knew I'd soon return to The City where I belonged.

But now, a year later, after cancer had taken over my life and imposed an expectation on him that he cow-towed to, the most common phrase spoken in my direction in all of 2012 was now coming out of the mouth of the one person I was least expecting it to. Valentine.

"This isn't working."

In a rickety, bargain bin hotel room in Dayton, Ohio he was setting my brain ablaze with the notion that he no longer wanted to be together. Just days before he was wooing me with sweet nothings, which evidently was all they were, nothing. Just days ago, he was telling me that he was looking for jobs in The City for when all of this cancer business was over and done with so we could move in together. Days ago. Not weeks or months ago where there was wiggle room for change of heart, not weeks or months ago where the chemotherapy charging through me would have scrambled his intentions over time in my brain, but literally days in which the hours could have been counted.

I was face down on the faded floral pattern comforter shrouded bed hugging the single hotel issued crinkly pillow listening to him stammer through his poorly rehearsed speech. His words didn't even seem like they were his, but this far into the game, nearly a year to date since we met, in the same town we met in, he was slowly chipping away at the false trunk of a relationship that I'd began to feel as if though I somehow fabricated. I couldn't even look at him. I stared at the floor watching his size sixteen sneakers beat the dust out of the brown carpet as he paced. Was that carpet supposed to be brown, or was it just that filthy?

Eventually Valentine sat on the bed next to me and put his big hand on my back right between my shoulder blades.

"Are you going to be ok?"

He always gave himself too much credit. Of course, I was going to be ok, maybe not now, maybe not tomorrow, but I'd be fine. Still, with radiation coming to a close, my underarm still raw and scabbed with black, burnt tissue, formerly skin, and an allogenic stem cell transplant looming before me, it all began to sink in that I was scared. Petrified. More so now then I was an hour ago, because now I was alone. Sure, Mother and Father, and my sisters, and friends were a constant in my situation, but this was different. None of them could promise me a future after all of this was over, and that's what I was clinging to: a future, of any kind. They all were there for me, and going to be, and I knew that, but not in the way Valentine had promised.

Valentine's giant hand covered the entirety of my shoulders, rubbing the nape of my neck. It took me a second, but the reality of what just happened, the one-sided conversation I listened to, set in and I began to cry. I buried my face in this sad excuse for a pillow and began to openly and violently weep, cleansing myself of the lies, the travel, the long-distance bullshit, the deception, the betrayal. Even the mice in the walls silenced their scurrying for a moment.

"What am I going to do?"

Non-verbally, covered in mucus, and as nodesy as possible, I let it out; I let it all out, Viola Davis style. What was I going to do? Not once had I faced this alone, alone as in single, since day one of this disaster. Not once. Finally, I had gotten to a point where I felt relatively back to my old self again, and elevated because, congratulations Edward, for the first time in four years, you've landed a boyfriend. Now all of that was gone. Even though he sat right next to me in silence, and I laid there face down in a mental void, more upset at the non-plan, non-future ahead of me, he was gone.

It only took a few minutes for me to calm myself down. Valentine sat there like a lump staring at the floor while I was curled up in a ball. His complacency grabbed my attention and I suddenly stopped crying. I was shocked at how quickly that made me stop crying; the sight of him sitting there, not moving, not reacting, seemingly not caring.

"Ugh. Ok. Now what?"

He was still in the hotel room. I wanted him out. I wanted to leave as well. I needed to take a walk. Wounded as I was, I was sure I could find it in me to get changed into clothing I'd wear in public and walk out the door, one foot before the other.

"I told Marta we'd meet her for drinks."

What? You were going to break up with me and then celebrate with your sister and me? Seriously? Cool. Hoisting myself off the bed, I walked past Valentine and over to the hotel bathroom. I closed and locked the door and squared off to the sink, placing my hands on the sides of it for support. I was so mad at myself. I looked at that guy in the mirror and felt genuine disappointment in him for being such a gullible fool. This whole week I'd spent time with friends with whom I had done Hairspray and were local to the area, telling them how great things were going with Valentine and how I would consider moving there if he couldn't find a job in The City. That we had talked about marriage and kids and future stuff. Gullible. Stupid. Ridiculous.

Had I completely kidded myself into thinking that any of this was real? Had cancer and the rigors of its treatment needed a distraction? Had cancer selected the biggest distraction it could think of? It's fine. It's fine. It's all fine. Splashing some water on my face and giving the man in the mirror one last side eye, I re-entered the room where Valentine stood by the door waiting for me.

"You don't have to go if you don't want to."

Oh, no. I was going. I was definitely going.

Valentine crossed the bar to the bathroom leaving me alone with his sister, Marta. I was drunk and underfed, and definitely not in the best of headspaces. I didn't really feel like talking. Marta and I stood along a banister in the very crowded bro-bar scanning the room during a break in conversation.

"Are you ok? These things happen."

At first, I thought she meant cancer, to which I replied that, all things considering, I was going to be fine; there was a plan. About halfway through that statement, and my bourbon and ginger ale, I realized she didn't mean cancer at all and actually meant that her stupid, big, little brother had ended it. Straw in mouth, I considered clarifying, retracting my sentiment, and giving her the real answer, which was that over the course of the evening my sadness had turned from hurt to fear, and I was terrified to go back to The City. There was a buffer between this break up and my return to New York, because I was headed to Fort Lauderdale in the morning to visit my sister, Crissy. I refrained and just let her think that I was a wall of strength, and had already moved on, and was fine, but I was not.

Drunker, and back in my shithole of a hotel in the colon of Ohio, I stumbled through the door and flung my shoes off my feet as I continued walking further into the room. Each kelly-green boat shoe hit the wall and fell, defeated, onto the hideous brown carpet. Valentine had driven me back after nearly falling asleep standing up at the bar. It was time to go, and it was time to GO!

"Do you want me to stay or do you want me to go."

Go. I wanted him to go. But my newfound, bourbon-fueled fear of life and things to come had taken over. The last thing I wanted was to be in a rank hotel room in the middle of nowhere, where my chances of being hacked to bits by a crazy redneck with a chainsaw were arguably much higher than usual.

"Can you please just sleep next to me with your arms around me one last time?"

It sounded so timid coming out of my mouth. I almost felt ashamed that I had even asked, but I figured 'why not'?

"If that's something you need."

Fuck you! Valentine's big arms were wrapped around my torso like a boa constrictor. The heat from his body was only somewhat lulling me to sleep as my brain drunkenly burned through our evening. No matter the amount of alcohol pumping through me, every time I could feel my body slipping into the quietness of sleep, I'd awake at the realization that this person holding on to me didn't want to be there. He no longer wanted me in his life. Stubborn as I am, I stood firm in my request, and laid there watching the headlights from the highway shift the shadows of the curtain from one side of the room to the other.

Morning finally came, and with an urgency that only a hangover could fuel, Valentine drove me to the airport in silence, without any coffee in my blood stream. We left hours before my flight so he could get to work on time. Evidently Old Navy was cracking the whip on tardiness. He pulled my bags out of the trunk of his rickety car in the drive-up next to the departures gate at Dayton International Airport. I stood there watching him put the canvas weekender on the sidewalk next to my feet. The same bag I packed time and time again for my extended overnight stays at the hospital, and the same bag I packed time and time again for theatre contracts.

He stood on the drive, me on the sidewalk, and for a moment we were eye level.

"So..."

Valentine went in for a hug. I stood there, still, with his arms around me fighting the urge to throw my arms around his thick neck and cry. He grabbed and squeezed me into him, and almost by reflex, I forgot my stance, and returned the hug. His sway really had me. Pulling out of the hug, his lips hesitantly made their way onto mine, and I tried to pull back. I scrunched up but proved to be too weak to resist after a night of interrupted sleep. I let it happen. I wanted it to happen.

He walked away, headed for the driver's side door of his jalopy. He was walking away. This was it. This was maybe the last time I was going to see him.

Fighting the anger and frustration I was feeling, I picked up my bag and turned my back on his car as he folded himself inside.

"Don't look back, Edward. Keep it together, and don't. look. back."

Walking into the airport, through the automatic doors, into the terminal, I fought with the magnetic pull that was trying to turn my head around for one last look at him. My heart hurt, and my gut was twisting into knots, but the rumble of his motor faded away, and I knew I was safe. I was safe and could check in for my flight.

I sat in the waiting area at my flight gate watching planes come and go. There was still a good three or four hours until mine was even going to board, and I began to question if I could tolerate hanging around that long. Just simply being in this town made me nauseated. Heavy as I felt, I pushed myself off the plastic chair and walked up to the attendant at the terminal podium. Hoping there was an earlier flight I could take; I took out my wallet.

"There is one boarding in about 20 minutes."

Great. Get me out of here. The circulated air of the terminal was gagging me with both hands, on top of the suffocating concept of being dumped, alone, and unsure how to move forward, on top of the anxiety of cancer. Though there was still progress with radiation, though my hair had begun to grow back, I anxiously dropped the seventy-five-dollar flight-change fee to get the hell out of dodge. Yes, I would still have to wait for my connecting flight to Fort Lauderdale on an extended layover in Chicago, but at least I'd be the fuck out of Ohio.

"How do you feel?"

Dr. Aurora interrupted the fresh wound I'd zoned-out into. Unintentionally she kicked the lid off the pot I was so anxiously trying to keep closed and asked about the literal straw that had caused me to seek out a mental health professional in the first place, personal life.

I tried, I really tried to brush it off as 'oh brother', but that proved to be an impossibility. I didn't even answer her. I moved my feet on to the floor, so they were flat on the carpet and put my coffee down on the windowsill. I tucked my lips inside my mouth, lowered my chin into my chest, and sat there shaking. How dare she bring that up. Bracing myself on the front of the cushions, holding onto them as though I were wringing my ex's big, stupid neck, I held every part of my body together with a deep breath. It was time to cut the crap and play by the rules.

"You asked how I felt. Lost. I'm lost."

And I sure was. Mostly I meandered from waiting room, to exam room, to taxi, to home. Any interruption in that routine was an abnormality and special circumstance. If I wasn't at Grizabella's bar getting shit-faced on bourbon and ginger ale doubles, I was at home doing the same, or burying myself in Netflix. I'd become a shell, a zombie with no compass, no navigation whatsoever, and no direction that wasn't Manhattan County Hospital. My brain seemingly hadn't caught up with my reality yet. It had taken over so quickly that I constantly felt out of control, and so, being out of control was how I had regained control over my life.

The oversized sack of shit I decided to dedicate and waste a year of my life to had broken up with me to be with someone who looked as if their face had been stitched on by a Hollywood villain's make-up artist. It had recently come to light that he was dating someone else nearly the whole time we were together. I was furious, but what does one do in that position? Continue to date someone because they have cancer? Submit to being a pity-boyfriend? I gave into the possibility that maybe I didn't blame Valentine, and I hated myself for it. I also hated him for it.

The phrase 'having the rug ripped out from under you' seemed like the only way that I could explain myself, and like the palest comparison I could muster. A carpet? Not a carpet: my whole fucking life. My whole fucking existence had been ripped out from under me. Every ounce of identity I ever had, from physical to professional, disintegrated right before my eyes in a matter of days, hours in some cases, and I never allowed myself to acknowledge that fact. I wanted Disney happiness around me at all times.

No crying allowed. No gloom and doom; just cocktails, and Netflix, and family, and friends. Glazing over the severity of this downward spiral only got me so far until, here I was, sitting in a therapist's office shaking and sobbing like someone had just severed my arm without a numbing agent. In a way they had. I was stuck, unable to move, unable to make choices for myself; simply going along with whatever the doctors were telling me. Going along. Following. Going along. Letting each and every treatment molest and violate me in demeaning and indecent ways.

Maybe I needed this couch? Maybe I needed Dr. Aurora!

"How do you feel?"

I wanted to leave New York. Nothing felt like home anymore, and the reason I had moved to The City in the first place was so far in the distance I could barely even remember what that reason was. Any savings I had accrued on the road was now squandered on medical bills and frustration. The few mini vacations that I had taken to South Florida to visit Crissy, though resulting in medical complications every single time, had struck a chord leaving me considering the possibility of relocating closer to a beach. It had become my new happy place, escape.

In a cab on the one hundred-block journey downtown to Dr. Aurora's office, I rode with my head out the window of the taxi like a dog. It was far too cold to tolerate the temperature outside, but the cool air on my face was like cutting it, it made me feel alive. As Riverside Park and The Hudson River whizzed by, my Zillow app open and searching Fort Lauderdale apartments, a familiar color palette caught my eye. Manhattan Mini-Storage in all of its purple, white, and orange glory saved my life in a single advertisement.

"Remember: If you leave The City, you have to live in America."

What was I fucking thinking? I sat in the cab chuckling to myself, at my silliness of ever considering leaving. This had been my home for the entirety of my adult life. I was lucky enough to work as a full-time actor experiencing other parts of the country. There were parts that were lovely, and not so lovely, but the reality of leaving my home to go live in those places permanently was not something that was going to work for me. I was regaining perspective with myself at every passing exit sign on the highway and I mentally unpacked my bags and began deleting the real estate apps I'd downloaded on my phone.

"How do you feel?"

Hurt. Disgusting. I knew what I looked like. I had a mirror. There was no fooling myself into believing I looked anything like my photo on the dating apps that I remained on for validation; reaching and fishing for someone to tell me that they thought what my former self looked like was desirable. What little hair was left on my head was silky uneven spots of peach fuzz. My facial hair, if any, was patchy and oily. My body was bloated and floppy in a way I hadn't experienced since I was shopping for jeans in the husky section of the department stores as a kid with grandma. I barely had a whisper of eyebrows left.

Anytime I did decide to meet up with someone, I could see their faces force steadfastness, fighting the desire to contort and wonder what the hell they were looking at, what was this thing.

First it was a tall, beefy photographer slash actor that met me at Grizabella's bar in the Upper West Side on my invitation and whooped and hollered along with the girls but sat as far away from me as possible and ignored me the entire time. After a few drinks, he couldn't have gotten out of there faster. I knew why. Then it was a muscled up Spanish guy in Washington Heights who came over and went through the motions of my proposed tryst, but afterwards asked me how long I had been sick as I collapsed, nearly blacking out on the bed, heaving in oxygen.

"What? Sick? I'm fine."

Evidently his roommate at one point 'looked just you.' I couldn't get him out of there faster.

Dr. Turner had given up on chemo and moved me onto radiation.

"There are two kinds of Non-Hodgkin's: Chemo sensitive, and radiation sensitive."

Unsure why it had taken four rounds of unsuccessful chemo over the course of three months to bring this up or do something about it, I was relieved for the change. I saw my radiation technician every day. Monday through Friday at 5:30pm I'd make my way to Manhattan County Hospital and lay on their big metal bed for a few minutes to be inundated.

Dr. Molina, studious and quirky, had become a recent regular part of my life. He made me feel welcome and comfortable enough on his giant nuclear slab to open up to him. Soon, he started prompting conversation sprouting beyond 'how are you today?' and 'hold still!' to a point where I began to compulsively talk, justifying who I was as a person before Seymour took hold.

After an appointment, I showed him my headshot. The one I'd used not months before that booked me all of my work. Once the image popped up on my phone, I turned it around and showed him the old me.

"Oh, my god! THAT'S YOU?!"

Taken aback, I nodded and put my phone back in the gown pocket. Had I really fallen so far away from this headshot that it was inconceivable that it could possibly be me?

"Yup. It was."

Changing back into my street clothes from the starchy hospital gown, I looked at my naked body in the full-length mirror. Hairless. Sloppy. All the things I hadn't accepted yet became clear as day in that mirror.

I immediately went home and fired up a dating app or two, angrily looking for anything but a date. Using old photos that didn't reflect my current self, I tried to regain control; make myself feel better about myself. No hat, no pair of shoes, no number of cocktails could heal this one. I was not equipped to know how to translate my old body and circumstances into my new ones. The words of Dr. Molina kept echoing in my ear with each response I'd get for my year-old photos. I began to line them up: Marcos, Esteban, a line of Orderlies. One by one, by two, by one they all came over and took their turns under the Christmas lights. Deep inadequacy raged through me, and I found myself angry that I didn't know how to deal with this, and that this is how I chose to try. How was I supposed to navigate this new territory with my balls cut off?

One of the arrivals buried his face in the pillow next to mine so he didn't have to look at me while he did his business. I was gutted. Lying there nearly in tears as he grunted and forced his way to a finish, I pushed it down. I pushed it all down. As he got dressed, he avoided eye contact, and walked out of the apartment before even putting his shirt fully on. It was awful, but still, I continued to open the door for each ticket taker, and we proceeded to use each other for our own selfish needs.

"How do you feel?"

I was not ok.

1.14 Everything's Coming Up Roses

Radiation replaced chemo as a last-ditch effort since nothing else was working. Seymour kept shrinking, and growing back, and shrinking, and growing back, but had finally stopped with the onset of radiation. It seemed to be working. I liked radiation, as much as one could. It was quick, easy, and didn't make me feel like regurgitated garbage run over

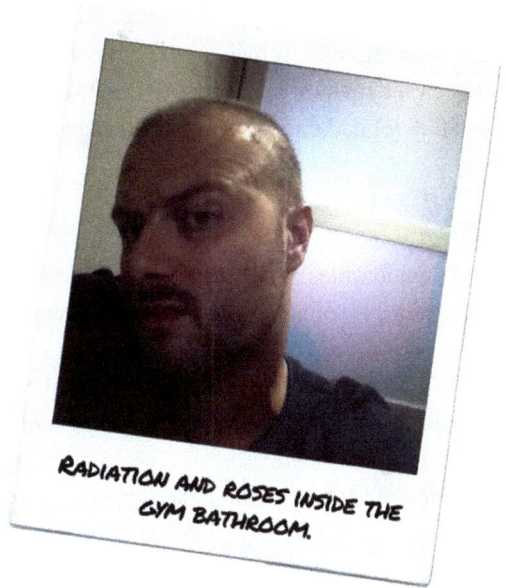

RADIATION AND ROSES INSIDE THE GYM BATHROOM.

twice. It wasn't perfect, but it was a welcome change. Besides, I'd have traded the side effects of chemo for those of radiation any day; fatigue and constipation verses perpetual clamminess, chemo brain, weird food cravings leading to barfing, hormone bloat, and insanity? Yes please. It gave my body a break for repair. I could walk farther, do stairs, and grow hair. Though perpetually anxious of the outcome, as this was the final option before the 'bring you to death and back; Stem Cell Transplant', I could at least get some footing on life again.

Columbus Circle whirled the sullen remains of fallen leaves from the autumn months before around. The perpetual crust of the city swirled into the air on, what felt like the blusteriest day of March there had been. The crosswalk signs flashed with warning that soon the Yellow Cabs revving their engines would unapologetically mow you down lest you remove yourself from their devil's path. My foot landed on the sidewalk as a downtown bound taxi swished through the cross walks nearly clipping my heel. Readjusting the strap of my bag over my shoulder forging onward to West 55th Street where I was to face an old, now unfamiliar friend: My gym.

As I approached the front door an all red "T" was plastered on the wall outside of the main door where a different logo used to hang. What happened? Removing my mirrored aviator glasses in disbelief to get another look, I walked through the door only to find that the color scheme had completely changed from white and light green to red and more red. Yonkers, the front desk attendant, who was also not the usual, took my gym pass and swiped it, slowly handing it back. His face froze looking at the screen twice and then me, confused at the discrepancies between the man on the computer, and the thing in front of him. It was me, but it wasn't. A lot had changed since that photo had been taken.

"Hi, welcome to Toreadorables."

Toreadorables? Are you fucking kidding me? What the hell kind of name for a gym is that? It sounded like a beauty pageant for toddlers. I hated it.

"We took over the old gym, but don't worry, your membership is still the same, I just need you to sign this form stating I told you about the merger."

I signed some papers. What the hell was this? I get cancer and leave for four months and suddenly my gym has gone from Midtown Broadway gay Mecca to a fratty meathead factory? Passing the desk and entering the memory of a gym I used to attend, I felt like I was entering an alternative universe version of my gym rather than a new one.

The layout was all the same: cardio machines on the left wall in three rows facing the weight machines, facing the free weights. The black pleather upholstery on the weight machines had been changed to the same red of the 'T' outside. All I wanted was the comfort of my old gym. All I wanted was to return to my gym, work out in familiar territory, and feel like myself again. Instead, what I got was a divide of new members who looked like a weightlifting competition, and the lost, stripped, blank faces of the previous members who were pumping iron looking as confused and terrified as I felt to be back.

I took in a breath of the gym bag air. Whatever. The space doesn't matter. I made it here in the first place, and that's half the battle right now. So, I put my bag on the floor behind an elliptical and mounted it. My first time back and I already felt accomplished; I was such a boss on that elliptical. My feet began to push against the resistance I was timidly edging upwards testing my new limitations when I noticed the cardio corner looking at me. Looks and shocked sneers darted my way as if I were some sort of creature from beyond as I glided up and down.

"I shouldn't be here."

The stares of the neighboring fitness fiends started the rotation of the frustration hamster ball I was now treading. No, I shouldn't be here, agreeing with the on-lookers.

Gyms are filthy, germ-infested places, but now, off the chemo and onto daily radiation, I wasn't fatigued after a shower, I wasn't crippled after making breakfast, so determined was I to be active, be aggressive towards my recovery. Even if that meant pushing the envelope, even if that meant risking getting sick with no immune system left, I was going to go back to my church and work. But now I was questioning all of that, and the more I became out of breath from a mere three minutes of light cardio, the more I felt pressed to leave. Chemo brain began to dominate in the eyes of the spectators trying to gauge what was wrong with me. Familiar faces of the fitness regulars searched my face as I bounced up and down, trying to confirm the notion that they recognized me from somewhere, but I didn't want them to.

I began to feel less than well as I pushed onward, but I wasn't stopping. I was going to do this if it killed me. I had become a spectacle, like an exhibit at the zoo. Behind my uniform of an oversized zip-up hoodie and a skullcap I hid pushing myself forward to work out, to finish the ten-minute cardio goal I had set for myself. I blocked out what I could of the gym with a soundtrack of Kelly Clarkson and Broadway. What doesn't kill you just makes you fat and hairless, at least in my circumstances.

As I defied gravity on the elliptical, my heartbeat raced in sporadic syncopation against the tempo of Stephen Schwartz. I imagined I was on the steps of the palace actively pursuing the pitch smeared steps heading away from The Prince, or cancer, or whatever, I wasn't sure, but somewhere up or down the flight, my feet stuck.

After only seven minutes of pumping my legs to the beat of the Great White Way and American Idol royalty, I dismounted the machine-like Snow White's prince dismounting his white steed. Cardio always was my least favorite thing in the world to do, until hospital stays became a thing, and then cardio became my second least favorite thing in the world to do. So, I stopped. I picked up my bag, nearly dropping it through my exhaustion and its now seemingly heavier disposition, I walked across the back of the room behind the cardio machine heaving and holding onto the wall, only tripping on my own two feet once. I bent over the water fountain lapping up the tiny trickle of barely cold water that came out of it making a game plan in my head of what I was going to do next, if I could do anything next.

Chest. That's easy. I'll do chest. My breath came back as I slowly, discreetly walked down to the bench press making sure no one was using it. The gym wasn't that full, but I still wanted to make sure I didn't have to come in contact with anyone while I was there, afraid I'd see someone I actually knew. Not wanting to hurt what was left of my ego, or myself, I grabbed two twenty-five-pound disks, each heavier than the next as I lined up the spoke with the hole in the weight to secure it onto the bar. Lying down on the bench, I evaluated the bar and tried to take a mental scan of my upper body to make sure I was lined up correctly as to avoid dropping weights on myself. One of my biggest fears has always been dropping a press bar on my face, not that, at this point, it would have made much of a difference to my appearance anyway.

Alright, deep breathe in, engage core, and one, two, three, push. The bar levitated above my body at the end of my arms, and I mentally prepped myself for its descent upon my chest.

One.

So far so good.

Two.

Alright, I think I got this.

Three.

My stomach started to turn at each lowering of the bar. The engagement of my core to the inertia of the press seemed to have caused quite the stir around my insides.

Four.

Ok, that's enough. I need to go. And by go, I mean off this bench, across the room, and sprint to the men's room. The bar slammed back against the frame and the whole gym turned around to see if someone was being decapitated under the weight of their false over achievement. I grabbed my bag, clenching my innards as each foot landing on the ground provoked more gravity and urgency to move inside and out.

Dodging the other fitness pursuers and their flailing equipment I clumsily slumped, staggered, and galloped across the gym floor frantically towards the lights of freedom and release of the men's locker room. Praying as I darted past the receptionist that my bowels wouldn't unleash themselves for another thirty seconds. The heat in my stomach began to swell, burn, and push as I flashed an attempted smile at Yonkers, a smile that likely looked more like I was having a stroke or was mid-cry than an actual grin.

Oh God, what is HAPPENING? My lower abdomen felt like a big foot was standing on it, pushing so hard that my back started to ache and cramp. I think my breathing stopped all together as to not shatter my midsection any more than the contact my feet were making with the floor would.

Christ, don't shit on the floor. Christ, don't shit on the floor!

FUCK! DO. NOT. SHIT. ON. THE. FLOOR!

Somewhere within the span of internally cursing myself into a shame hole where I wouldn't shit on the floor, and triathelon-ing to the toilet, thrashing through reception, I remembered radiation. One of the common side effects was constipation, and now that the concept had raced to the forefront of my mind, and the forefront of my back door, and the fires of hell were about to come spewing out of me, it occurred to me that I hadn't gone to the bathroom in that capacity for a number of days. A concern I seemingly overlooked, as I was a morning regular, and probably would have gone twice by noon. It was now 4pm. The last I remembered fixing this problem was on Monday. It was now Thursday, and an hour and a half before my next radiation appointment and I wasn't entirely sure, now, that what was about to happen was going to get me there on time.

Praise the saints, there was an open stall: the middle one. I body checked the door open and didn't even lock it before shoving my gym shorts down around my thighs; there wasn't enough time to make it to my ankles. I'd worry about that later. No sooner had I made contact with the plastic and porcelain seat, then what seemed like twenty-five-years' worth of meals rapidly and unapologetically burst their angry way out. A raining from the do-it-yourself Niagara Falls beneath me soaked my underlings, the sound of which, I'm sure, reverberated and traveled far beyond the stall, into the lobby, onto West 55th Street and Ninth Avenue, and into space itself. The pain, the humiliation, the ridiculousness and humor of the whole situation; I was a puddle of emotions, in a puddle of postmortem feelings I had eaten, and they just wouldn't stop.

Like a broken Play-Doh factory, I sat there heaving outwards. My body contorting against my control, making sure nothing was left; Making sure that I would never be motivated to eat ever again as the continuous, never-ending stream of shame furiously exited my body. I had now resorted to bracing my arms against the walls of the bathroom stall as leverage to assist in my bearing down, simultaneously trying to remain as non-vocal as possible. Grunting and yelping in a men's room is never really smiled upon, especially in a gym in Hell's Kitchen, or maybe except in a gym in Hell's Kitchen.

Desperately screaming in silence begging my bowels for a cease-fire, panting for an end to even be remotely in sight, I sat there flushing every few minutes, pretending that no one was nearby, and no one could share in the redolence I was emitting, but at long last, twenty minutes in, seven flushes total, and ab workout complete, my penance had finally come to a close. I sat with my hands on my knees, bent over looking at the floor watching the sweat drip off the tip of my nose into my gym shorts that stretched from ankle to ankle.

"Well, that was fucking awful."

I remained seated a top the loo, anticipating a second round I couldn't imagine existing considering the two hundred pounds of sorrow that just evacuated the dance floor. I grasped for the single ply toilet paper, of course it had to be single ply, and three rolls later, I was finally able to retire from the throne and hoist my shorts to their original locale.

Fumbling with the slide lock on the stall door, I almost felt bad touching it in the first place, I shoved the door open and stumbled over to the sink to sterilize my now putrid hands. With barely any soap left in any of the dispensers, I cursed myself for not bringing bathroom toiletries. Of course, the one-time I don't bring soap to shower is the one time I desperately needed it.

Returning to the stall to grab my bag, the smell of hate still in the air wafting around, I snatched the bag off the floor and flung it over my left shoulder. I turned around and looked at myself in the mirror, seeing the reflection I had ignored while vigorously washing my hands.

"Woof."

I immediately rushed the sink and turned the cold water on, bending down to splash some on my face in hopes of cleansing me of the battered woman look I was sporting. Should one have been able to compare my face and my now ruined backside, I'm not sure which would have been in better shape at the moment. Snatching a fist full of paper towels, I dabbled and rubbed my face dry, exfoliating, searching for something that looked like me when I walked in the door; something less pale and ashamed. A tireless vain effort, I gave up and walked out of the men's locker room and back into the lobby. Briskly and casually stepping lightly as to not draw attention to myself, remaining a casual part of the minor traffic hovering around the front desk, but to no avail. They knew. They smelled, they saw, they knew.

Edward Miskie

1.15 Get Out and Stay Out

Back at Manhattan County Hospital once again, I paced back and forth between the orange biohazard trash bin and the door. I was getting up the nerve to stand my ground and tell Dr. Turner that I was done. The appointments, the cab rides, the depression, the fucking terrible port flushes that made me want to absolutely vom, the social anxiety, the blood transfusions, the constant paranoia I'd contract C-Diff or pneumonia were all

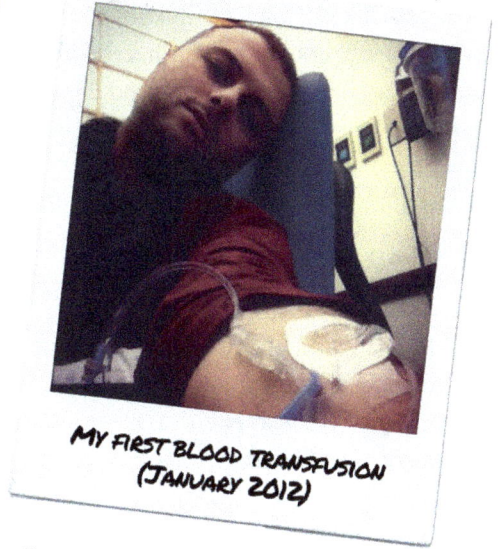

MY FIRST BLOOD TRANSFUSION
(JANUARY 2012)

about to be in the past. I had seen myself with hair once again, a glimpse of the man I was, and I wasn't going back. If the radiation was working, then there was no need for anything else. Right? Why do more chemo if there wasn't use for it; it wasn't working.

Something had shifted within me. The thirty days of daily radiation had turned my underarm black and red. It was totally raw, burned whenever I touched it, and was crusted over in black scabs that would often flake off into the gauze pad I taped over it. Though aesthetically horrifying, as if I were proof that the Walking Dead was a thing, Seymour began to disappear, to shrink. It seemed to be a success of sorts; the first success I had experienced in months. For the first time Seymour wasn't growing back.

I was motivated again. Despite everything else, I felt great, or at least a version of great! If I wasn't actually back to being a real person, I at the very least I was beginning to feel like one.

THANKS RADIATION?

So, now here I was in this cookie-cutter hospital room under a malfunctioning white strobe light waiting for Dr. Tuner. I was in a hurry to get this appointment over with. It felt uncomfortable. It felt weird. It felt like another break-up. Only this time, I was the one doing the breaking-up.

I sat down on the exam table and settled on staring at the doorknob, willing the doctor, a nurse, anyone, to walk in. My feet dangled over the edge of the table, slightly swinging back and forth, crinkling the white tissue paper beneath me. My ankles crossed swinging like a pendulum of a small clock keeping track of the passing time. I sat there in the loudest silence imaginable, with only the tissue paper under me as white noise. My thoughts glossed over my surroundings as I reviewed my game plan for when Dr. Turner did finally show up.

"Stick to your guns. Say no. You are allowed to say no."

Mid-way through my self-pep-talk, the abrupt peeling open of the door, a shattering cracking as if it were hermetically sealed to its frame, yanked me back into the room. Dr. Turner entered the room closely followed by Nurse Doralee. I had almost grown to nearly enjoy our visits together. But, by visits, I mean appointments in which she would tell me that nothing was going according to plan, and we would have to go back to the drawing board; literally, every single time. Through the gloomy news, we would find ways to laugh, and crack jokes at each other. It was a sick, fucked up, backwards enjoy ability. She shook my hand. Had we not graduated to hugs at this point yet? Doralee went into the corner and stood quietly, observing, and Dr. Turner sat herself down at the desk.

"We need to talk about this Stem Cell Transplant."

From the beginning, this transplant was a looming shadow that was acknowledged but never really discussed, and prognosis and the forecast of things to come were never actually clear.

"Basically, we kill your system with as much chemo as it can handle, and then inject a new system, bringing you back from 'death'."

That was the trajectory for May and June 2012 that Dr. Turner kept pushing and pushing. It sounded fucking terrible. It's why I was saying no.

Every time we had this transplant conversation it was one sided. Dr. Turner wanted me to have an Allogenic Stem Cell Transplant instead of an Autologous Stem Cell Transplant. Allogenic is when someone else is your Stem Cell donor. You are literally injecting someone else's juices into your body to replace your own after they've been evaporated by the highest dose of chemo your body could possibly handle before it kills you. This type of transplant, if, and only if, it works, fucks your life up permanently.

Someone else's DNA print is graphed into your body, your system recognizes it as a foreign object and can spontaneously reject it at any moment. It could be in the hospital, it could be five years after treatment, it could be at any moment it chooses. For this reason, you take an immunosuppressant for the rest of your life as a way of preventing your old system from puking out the new one and leaving you with nothing.

An Autologous Stem Cell Transplant is when you use your own Stem Cells. It's safer, it's less likely to be rejected, it doesn't require life-long medication to keep you alive, and you don't have to sit around waiting for a donor match to pop-up.

Still, Dr. Turner pushed for the Allogenic. Dr. Turner decided to put feelers out for a Stem Cell donor match in the national database with no luck. Dr. Turner decided to send blood test kits to Crissy and Jeanie to have them be tested as Stem Cell matches. No match. Even though Autologous wasn't her choice, Dr. Turner decided to humor me and lock me in the hospital basement for four days, five hours at a time, to will Stem Cells out of my body. No luck, yielding just a fraction of what was needed for a successful Autologous Transplant. That route increasingly began to feel like a dead end, but no other scenarios were being presented. I felt bullied, being bossed around by someone who seemed to have blinders on, heading in one direction with no steering wheel

Leaving the exam table for some solid footing, I walked across the room as she continued. Doralee shifted from the corner where she stood over to the edge of the desk where Dr. Turner sat. From where I stood, where I literally stood, the need for all of this new treatment seemed thin.

"Find a Stem Cell match, do more chemo, have the Allogenic Stem Cell Transplant, do two courses of full-body radiation, and see what happens."

That full body radiation thing rubbed me the wrong way, too. I saw what localized radiation did to my skin, and I didn't want to face the reality of being a six-foot-four walking scab. I perched against the wall opposite of Dr. Turner with my arms crossed, listening to her go on as she sat at her computer pulling up my records. Nurse Doralee was watching my every move, almost silently cheering me on, encouraging me to speak up.

Dr. Turner, with her every word, kept pushing the donor option. Dr. Turner decided everything. Dr. Turner gave me no choice. Dr. Turner pushed me to the edge of my tolerance.

"No. I really don't want to do that."

Nurse Doralee tensed up against the corner of the desk, nearly smiling. Dr. Turner assured me it was the right course of action without even flinching. Dr. Turner assured me there was nothing else we could do. Dr. Turner reminded me that all the chemo options had been exhausted. Dr. Turner pointed out that radiation seemed to be working, but results of that would not be conclusive for several months. Dr. Turner pushed that an Allogenic Stem Cell Transplant was the only next step in the process.

"No, by 'I don't want to do that', I'm actually telling you I'm not doing that. No!"

Nurse Doralee leapt off the floor and cheered me on. Her enthusiasm landed her at my side holding my hand, communicating that it was okay to continue. Still propped up against the wall, trying to come off as relaxed and calm, my monologue of why I didn't want to go through with this dominated the room and Dr. Turner. Nothing about 'bringing your body to the point of death and then bringing it back again' sounded like anything I wanted to do. Transplants were harder and harsher than anything I had already experienced, and with that as a baseline, I rejected Dr. Turner's plan.

Dr. Turner shirked, searching for a response.

"Because that's the route I want to take."

That was the best she could come up with? So that was not the route I wanted to take, and for the first time since that first day of being put in the hospital, I said no. Nurse Doralee's grip on my hand tightened, assuring me that I was making the right move.

Dr. Turner and I had a silent exchange. Maybe she was searching my face for a sense of weakness to break and bend me to her plan. Maybe she was hoping that I was kidding, as I so often was. Whatever her thought process was, the vibes of not budging on the subject must have shot right through her because she didn't press the issue again. Instead, she turned to her computer, typed in a few things, and turned back to me.

"I'm going to refer you to a doctor I trained under for a second opinion."

She handed me a piece of paper with a name and phone number.

"Doctor Mame Anthony. She's at Sloan-Kettering."

Sloan Kettering? This whole time Dr. Turner told me that Sloan Kettering treated their patients as a number and not a person and that if I wanted personalized care instead of being part of a large machine, then I should stay where I was. I listened to that. I allowed that to deter me from seeking out a specialist and stay where Dr. Deuteronomy had banished me to in the first place. And now this very person who told me to avoid Sloan Kettering was sending me directly there. That was enough for me. The audacity to act against my best interest for whatever statistical gain there was severed any tie I had held on to with this place for the last few months.

Taking the piece of paper out of her hand in total disbelieve I was ready to get out and stay out. I was done. I let her know how I felt, and walked out, taking Nurse Doralee with me. I called her referral as soon as I left.

I was free, and I was going to Sloan Kettering; they'd understand me.

Edward Miskie

Act Two

21 It's Today

Back at Manhattan County Hospital once more.

"That'll be a $75 copy charge for your file."

I couldn't believe it. As if acquiring my biopsy samples, and medical files from Manhattan County Hospital for my voyage to Sloan Kettering wasn't difficult enough, Dr. Deuteronomy's office was now charging me for my medical

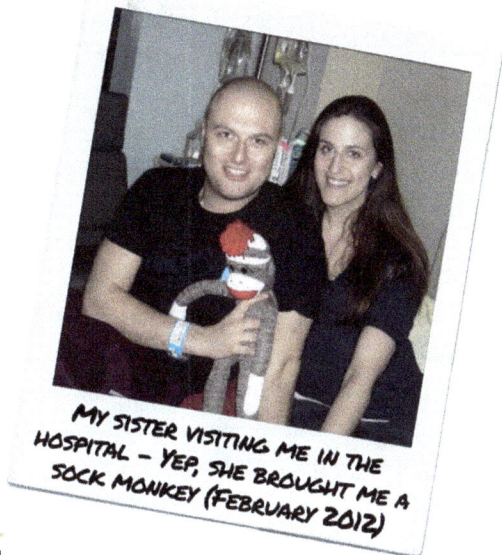

MY SISTER VISITING ME IN THE HOSPITAL – YEP, SHE BROUGHT ME A SOCK MONKEY (FEBRUARY 2012)

history of the last four years. Refusing to give them another cent, after having been charged $450 a pop for sixty-second hospital visits that included phrases such as:

"Are you sure they're giving you the right medication?"

"You look great."

"You've never looked better."

"They must be giving you soup instead of chemo."

I hung up the phone. Fuck that and fuck you. Sloan Kettering and my new doctor would just have to take my word on any questions they may have regarding my medical history.

Flinging my phone onto the bed in disgust, I sat down to tie up my shoes for my inaugural journey and appointment at the much-anticipated Sloan Kettering. Scooping up the plastic bag from the floor that contained the medical files and biopsy slides I did have, I headed for the door.

I marched through the 68th Street entrance of Memorial Sloan Kettering Cancer Center, independent, and about to be free. I whipped off my aviator sunglasses, my stride interrupted at the 'T' in the hallway, almost a casualty of doctor, patient traffic. I paused. I was already lost. The slick white floors, lit by rows of florescent lights, flanked by wood-panel walls, seemed like a maze filled with business. The shrill shriek of shoes skidding on the waxed floor sounded more like a basketball court then a hospital.

I decided on going left and ended up at a reception desk by the York Avenue entrance. From behind the console, the receptionist, Gooch, directed me where to go. Down the hall, left, then right, then left. What felt like practical joke directions, nearly expecting to end up in a trash room; I followed the hallways according to Gooch, and only got lost twice.

This waiting area, though adjacent to the hustle of the main hallways, somehow seemed off the beaten path, like I had stepped through The Wardrobe. Vera, the lone receptionist, handed me a clipboard and asked me to have a seat to fill out the attached novel sized workbook. I sat next to the water cooler and coffee maker, reading through the list of conditions I could have potentially had. No heart disease, no diabetes, no hepatitis, and no pregnancies. My circumstances began to pale in comparison. Sure, cancer wasn't great, but at least I wasn't pregnant and having insulin crashes and heart failures. Silver linings? I signed some papers. I checked on Seymour. Barely there! I got up and returned the lexicon of my health to Vera and sat back down to wait... and wait... and wait. The office was empty! How could this be taking so long?

"Edward Miskie."

Dr. Beauregard, the attending doctor in his dark blue scrubs, beckoned me over his glasses into the official Sloan Kettering doctor area. Distracted by his beard and demeanor, I nearly ran into the doorframe. Finally, an improvement in quality care already: hot staff members. If only things at Manhattan County Hospital looked this good before, maybe my life wouldn't have felt so bleak.

He directed me to an all-white room. The room felt pretty standard in my hospital experience, but there was something less institutional about it. Something welcoming? Was that the word? Less sterile? More sterile? I sat down in the chair by the desk, anticipating this new doctor's arrival. Not knowing what to expect of this person other than her name, I reviewed what I was going to say to her. Simply, I wanted to confirm, for my own peace of mind, that a transplant was a frivolous use of resources, and my time, and I was fine.

Over my left shoulder, the door flung open, and the smallest tornado of a woman I've ever seen walked in, piercing the linoleum floor with the spikes of her five-inch heels. Everything she was wearing looked like it was hand selected for her by Vogue. Dr. Mame Anthony! She was the head of the International Non-Hodgkin's Lymphoma board and top of the Sloan Kettering NHL pile. She was glorious, and terrifying. There was an energy that exuded from her that made me uncomfortable, but I immediately liked her at the same time. She nearly disappeared below my shoulders as I stood to shake her hand. Gracefully, she glided her way around me, ignoring my hand, and sat at the desk smoothing her hand over the thigh of her not-expecting-a-doctor-to-be-wearing-that skirt. I sat back down in awe like it was my first day in The City from a small town in a square state.

"So, what has been going on and why are you here?"

Direct! I like direct.

I told her everything. How Seymour just appeared one hot summer's day while I was lying out in my parent's backyard. How I found him in the shower. She scoffed at the Cat Scratch Fever diagnosis nearly as hard as I did. I walked her through the Reno situation with the ultrasound, and inability to get a biopsy while I was out there because of the tangled web of referrals and insurance networks. We briefly lamented about the broken medical system pre and post Obamacare, interjecting that I was grateful to have been put back on my parent's insurance plan just in the nick of time for this diagnosis to occur.

"If you're going to get cancer, those are the circumstances you'd want to be under."

I gave her the whirlwind version of each step in this exodus out of Cancertown: The needle biopsy, the four rounds of failed chemo, radiation, and how it seemed to have worked. How Manhattan County Hospital kept pushing treatments on me with which I was not comfortable. How after my sisters came up as non-matches for the transplant, my parents and I had looked into renewing passports and traveling abroad to Germany or Switzerland to seek out alternative options. How Valentine told me exactly what I wanted and needed to hear and bailed on me for some other guy, and lied, and lied, and lied, and lied.

Her vacant stare made me nervous. Instead of stopping, I pressed on, boring her with the unnecessary details of the last six months of my life.

The end of my relationship with Valentine was the launch pad for my state of mental unraveling. How I started ThereAreGiants.com in spite of my suggestion to

Valentine that he should be the one to take on the project; it would boost his amateurish career as a writer. How he told me that was a stupid idea, twice. How I felt empowered by the outlet of having taken it on myself. How my having started such a thing out of thin air had such a positive response. How it angered the hell out of Valentine.

Deep breathe.

"Ok, anyway, enough about him."

Dr. Anthony got a word in edgewise and asked if I had brought the biopsy samples that were requested from Manhattan County Hospital. Crinkling through the plastic bag on the floor, I pulled out a box. It looked like a Whitman's sampler. No one would have ever known that it contained glass slides of samples of my body on it; samples of cancer. For a moment, I was silent. I had finally stopped yammering on about my life for a minute and watched her open the packaging. Beyond the packing tape and the Styrofoam was the code to my cancer: just sitting there frozen in a slide. Dr. Anthony picked up one of the slides and held it to the light.

"Oh, that's not the kind of cancer you have."

Wait, what? How did you do that? You didn't even have a microscope to look at the slide under. Who is this woman? After all this time, after all of this bullshit my diagnosis was wrong? My mind began to rage and race against Dr. Turner. I was ready to call a lawyer and annihilate Manhattan County Hospital.

"Yeah, it's actually Rare Diffused Enlarged B Cell Non-Hodgkin's Lymphoma."

Stunned, I sat there looking at her in disbelief. What was going on? I couldn't tell if this was a better or worse scenario than the one, I had just removed myself from.

"Don't worry all the treatment is basically the same so at least we don't have to start over."

She paged through the list of medications I'd been put on. Stopping two or three prophylaxes down the list.

"They had you on BACTRIM during your stem cell collection?"

Yes, they did. Those big white horse-pill antibiotics that I was choking down? I was on them.

"No wonder you couldn't collect Stem Cells; Bactrim fucks with your blood counts."

I could have absolutely screamed. This new information began to poke holes in the wall of conviction I had walked in here behind. So, was the cancer gone? Was it still there? No! It wasn't still there; radiation took care of it. Seymour was shrinking more, and more each day. It was totally gone. Right?

Through my teetering stance with sanity, I sat as attentively and as relaxed as I could be. The last thing I wanted her to do was see that I was worried. I was still going to tell her 'no' to the transplant, but she was determined and convinced that there was no reason that I couldn't collect my own stem cells.

YES! SO WAS I! At long last, someone who at least understood where I was coming from as far as that was concerned.

"Who was your doctor there?"

I told her. Dr. Turner.

"Well, shame on her, I taught her better than that."

It was funny. Was it funny? I don't know. Maybe? I wanted to laugh-scream. I wanted to throw up. I wanted to find Dr. Turner and throw her under a bus. I wanted to throw something, maybe the cancer cell samples unwrapped on the desk. Instead, I took a deep breath and rebounded off this news and proceeded to explain why it didn't make sense to me for the Stem Cell Transplant to be a thing in the first place. Radiation had Seymour on a decline, blah, blah, blah, etcetera.

"Oh, no, you don't have to do the transplant... "

HA! I knew it! I knew I was right!

"...but you definitively won't live to see thirty if you don't."

Jesus. Fuck. Her statement knocked the wind out of me. I sat there looking at her. Thirty was only four and a half years away. Everyone has told me that thirty is a major turning point. Was my turning point going to be six feet under? Not wanting to let go of the 'no' stance I had so firmly taken with myself, I began to weigh what levels of risk I was willing to take to get out of doing this transplant. What was I willing to take on? A minute or so passed, and I inhaled coming-to from the brief coma I was in, processing my mortality.

This was my 'Drood' moment. My pick-your-own-ending. Whatever I said next was potentially going to impact my life in a major way. Like, as in, my life may come to an end at the end of either of these choices: No audience participation, no interactive voting to help me decide.

Dr. Anthony looked at me anticipating a reaction, any kind of recognition of comprehension of the magnitude of my situation.

"Like... you have a zero percent chance of living; in case you didn't understand."

Oh, I understood. I just couldn't think for a moment. Like an old sweater with a frayed yarn hanging off of it, I began to unravel the stitching I had sewn my 'no' to and let go.

"Well, then... I guess I'm doing the transplant."

Stunned, I sat there tuning out the next few sentences of protocol, experiencing flashbacks to my inaugural hospital check in, with day terrors of my life as an Avatar Cynthia Nixon. I came back down to the exam room. I was to have another needle biopsy to determine live cancer cells, which could potentially affect the success rate of the transplant. Then I was to have more chemo, and more Stem Cell collection.

"So, like... what are the chances of me dying anyway, if there are live cancer cells verses non-living cancer cells?"

She pulled up a flow chart from a database on her computer and scanned a few pages for information.

"Forty percent."

I guess that wasn't that high? I guess I could live with that statistic, literally. But I considered that forty percent, and Dr. Anthony's every day, dealing with this for however long she's been following this career path. Her entire adult life?

"How do you deal with all of this - all of this death?"

For a second, she went blank and shot a look at me away from the computer screen and her bank of information. I wondered if anyone had ever asked her that before.

"I put every case in a little box and file it away, WAY back in the back of my brain, and when I have time to deal with it, I do."

Knowing full well what her life must be like at the biggest cancer hospital in the country and basing what I had seen in the rippling hallways on my way over, I wasn't sure I bought that last part.

"Do you ever have time?"

Dr. Anthony went back to her computer and closed out the screens we had searched my query on.

"No."

As I left her office, I immediately felt the need for musical theatre therapy. I whipped out my headphones from my pocket and cued up Into the Fire from Scarlett Pimpernel. Retracing my steps from my arrival nearly two-and-a-half hours before, I strutted out onto East 68th Street, marching to the cadence of Frank Wildhorn. The song would end, and the automatic repeat feature would kick in giving me another wave of courage and hope.

Weirdly enough I didn't feel defeated. There was something about Dr. Anthony that carried my empowerment of leaving Manhattan County Hospital to this next chapter. Dare say that I was excited. I felt so at ease I could have run the entire way home. Occasionally bursting into song passing the unaffordable shops and boutiques of the East 60s, Douglas Sills and his effortless vocal fluidity pushed me through Central Park. I was 'that guy' that New Yorkers stare at and judge for their public emotional outbursts of incoherent rambling. Only my diction was perfect. I erupted out of the park at the Columbus Circle fountain and headed for the subway.

Floating through the tourists, and the sidewalks, and the unruly pigeons flocking towards the halal carts and hot dog stands, nearly getting annihilated by a taxi, I found myself bouncing down the stairs to the uptown A train. Finally, I trusted a medical professional in a way that I could let down my mental guard for a minute. Dr. Anthony put me at ease, which freed up some space in my head to acknowledge and appreciate the fact that I was relatively healthy, all things considering, single, and prognosis and plans were looking up. And even though there was definitely a downside, at the very least, in the end, if I survived the transplant, I would know I had made the right move. And with that wave of positivity, the first in ages, I got into the first car on the A train and stood in the window, watching the stations and support beams fly by as though I were the one flying.

22 Waving Through a Window

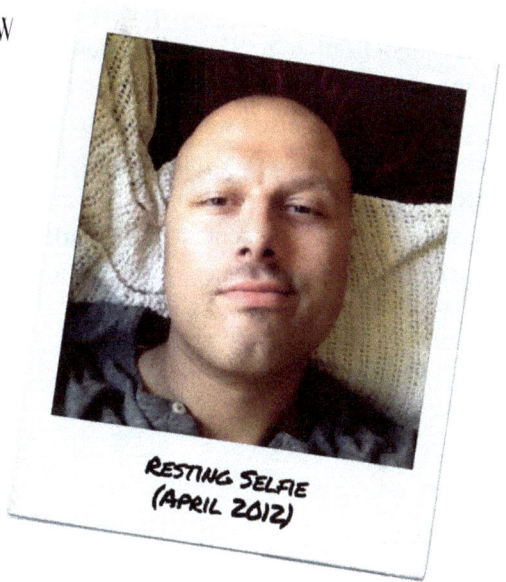

RESTING SELFIE
(APRIL 2012)

I had six days until my official Stem Cell Transplant check-in at Sloan Kettering to enjoy the Upper West Side: my new neighborhood. It was July 2012, a full year since Seymour had first popped into my life and my armpit. Since then, I'd lost friends, lost a boyfriend, lost my hair, endured four rounds of failed chemo, thirty days of radiation, a change in apartments, and a change in hospitals. But I was ok. I had plans.

I sat in the dark, my first night in my new apartment on West 73rd Street, with a bourbon in one hand, and a bag of freshly popped popcorn in the other. I had never lived in a building that faced another, giving light and windows into someone else's life. I watched the lights of the massive ornate building across the street pop on and off. My new neighbors were in perfect view, milling around their homes, unknowingly providing anthropological entertainment to hidden eyes. It felt so quintessentially New York. I got lost in my new neighbor's apartments.

Straight across the street from my apartment, there was a gay couple buzzing around their kitchen, bouncing back and forth between the table and the countertop taking turns preparing dinner, waiting for it to be done in the oven. Below them was a girl in her bed, barely moving, fading in and out of consciousness in the glow of her open laptop. Caddy corner to her, was an old man in a wheelchair sitting by the window just staring outside, wishing he could escape the prison his chair had become. A few floors up, a woman in her underwear doing side-bends, and standing leg raises as her late-night ab workout. I loved it.

This was going to be my new entertainment. I hadn't owned a television in nearly a decade. When I first moved to The City, I showed up with a twelve-inch boxy TV and a full cable and Internet package. I found most of my days were spent scavenging for jobs or exploring my new turf. So, having no money, I cancelled my cable, tossed out the TV, and instead, would find window seating in a random Starbucks, and watch people walk by. I'd make up stories of where they were going, who they were, what they were dealing with, but this was better. There was a calm about sitting in the dark, in silence, with only the tinkering of ice or crinkle of the popcorn bag cutting through my escape into someone else's story.

And someone else's story was exactly what I needed. I needed the stillness as a period at the end of a very long sentence of complications, bookended only by thin successes. I was about to plunge face first into this Stem Cell Transplant that scared the shit out of me. But content in my dark apartment with my cocktail and popcorn, I dove my way into each neighbor's home as I reflected on the doors and hurdles of the last six weeks.

221 This Had Better Come to a Stop

Dr. Marvin and Dr. Whizzer took turns ping-ponging between a microscope and me, collecting cell samples from the area where Seymour was. I was on an ebb and flow of nausea and anxiety as needles were punched into my left armpit; fourteen of them to be exact. All I wanted was a sliver of good news.

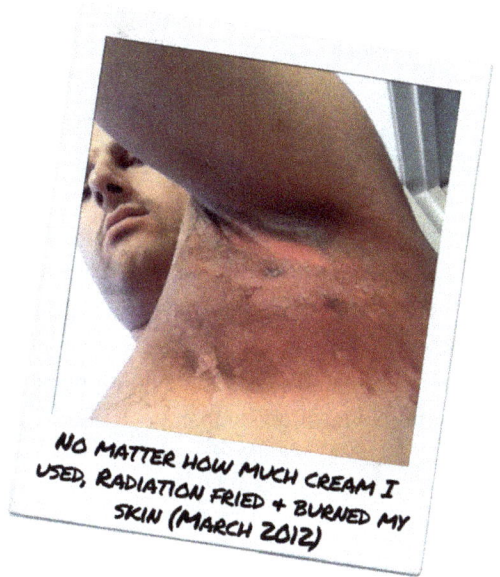

NO MATTER HOW MUCH CREAM I USED, RADIATION FRIED + BURNED MY SKIN (MARCH 2012)

Radiation had shrunk Seymour down to nearly nothing and there was suspicion that he was no longer alive. With weeks between my last radiation appointment and now, the only thing that had grown back was my hair, a shred of dignity, and self-confidence, so there was an assumed possibility that he was dead. His death was about to be determined. Now.

I laid there on the exam table under the blaring surgical lights, watching the javelin-sized needle balancing in Dr. Whizzer's gloved hand make its way over to my left axillary. Aiming for the heart of Seymour, my eyes were glued to my underarm with uncomfortable satisfaction. I wanted to look away, but I couldn't, and part of me was hoping to see the worst. Perhaps the needle would erupt what mass was left under my arm and blood, water, and fluids would spill all over the place. I was already so on edge facing the prospect that this could not go well that any gore would have paled in comparison to a negative report. If living cells were found, the transplant was going to be much more difficult, and I'd be less likely to survive.

With slick gusto and a flick of the wrist, the needle drove into my armpit like a tent stake, or something you'd secure a beach umbrella in the sand with. One after another, Dr. Marvin, and Dr. Whizzer took their turns maneuvering from the microscope across the room, both remaining nearly silent through my attempts at making painstaking small talk.

"Looks good. No living cells in this one."

Fourteen times. Fourteen nerve shattering times I awaited that sentence. I didn't celebrate either time. My focus, my balance on this fragile nerve I was on paralyzed me. I laid there in silence keeping my attentions on whichever doctor was at the microscope. Watching them. Analyzing their faces to try and predict what they were going to say, trying to beat them to the punch of telling me cancer was still present. I tried to translate each eyebrow, each tick, nuance, or breathe to see if I could guess what they were going to say before they said it.

One by one each slide came back clear, and even though that should have made me feel better and lighten my mood, it more so felt like I was honing in on a sentence; getting closer to the inevitable bad news I had, at this point, been trained and conditioned to expect. The buildup and the anticipation of this transplant translating over from Manhattan County Hospital to Sloan Kettering was all coming to a head right in front of my eyes; well, ears.

"And, done."

Finish line: crossed. Not a single cell had been found even remotely alive. Ding-dong, Seymour was dead. We did not feed the plant. As I walked out of the room, thanking Dr. Whizzer and Dr. Marvin, I felt just a little bit readier to take on this Stem Cell Transplant.

222 The Bend and Snap

Nurse Wyndham burst into my hospital room running in place, stretching, pulsing, and puttering around to an unheard beat. She made her way around my bed attaching my port to the appropriate poles, took my vital signs, and made sure everything was in place for the transplant prep chemo. Nurse Wyndham placed her pink, painted finger onto the pink, painted button on the fluids pump,

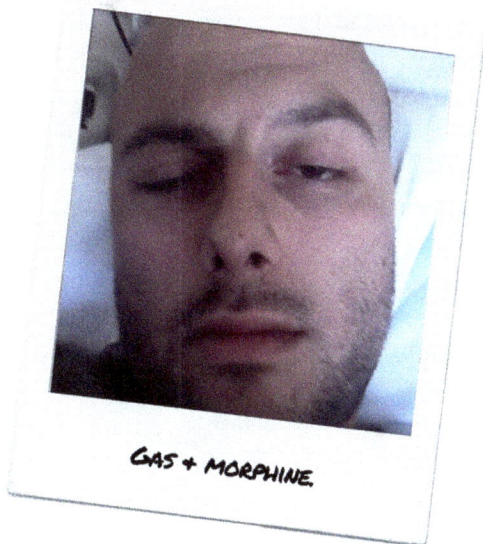

GAS + MORPHINE

commencing the flow of standard juices into my body. It was now time for her ab-buster class.

In a lightning speed reaction, I grabbed the sides of the bed and bent and snapped myself in half as pain and pressure wrenched its way across my abdomen. My side began to burn. Whatever it was built up so hard and so fast I struggled to inhale. As it worsened, I became convinced that something was going to rip out of my right oblique, split my side open, and do a cheer routine on the hospital bed. Mother sped over to the bed from the chair she had made herself comfortable in and took my left hand as I writhed around in pain, unable to breath or speak. What the fuck was happening?

Nurse Wyndham, without hesitation, produced a bag of morphine from her gym tote and hung up the bag on my IV pole.

"Exhale. And breathe, 2, 3, 4."

As the narcotic seeped into me, my face began to involuntarily scrunch, and my entire body began to itch and cramp.

"Oh! Are you allergic to morphine?"

Evidently, Nurse Wyndham, I was!

Bearing down with all the might I could stomach, through the max-out, side-sit-up series of doom, screams I couldn't phonate came out of my throat. My hands ached stubbornly holding grip to the bedrails waiting for it all to end, if it was ever going to. The excruciating and increasing pain swelled once again, and once again I tensed up so hard, I pulled the bed rail out of its socket.

As my personal chaos and commotion raged, Mother's eyes searched through her mental bible of medical explanations, her face blank and sheet white unsure if she was watching what would be the end of the DeltaNu hazing. In her conservative, calm, collected way Mother made a simple suggestion.

"Simethicone."

Nurse Wyndham dismissed the near benign medication as a ridiculous possibility, but to me the Gas-X made more sense than morphine, so I said yes. Or tried to say yes, which was more like a convulsing motion of my head that I was trying not to move in order not to upset the ravaging sorority in my side. Nurse Wyndham conceded. Through her fuss, not wanting to oblige, she informed us that we'd have to wait for her to call up the anti-gas medication from the pharmacy.

Another ab set took hold, and the focus of the room blurred. I couldn't see. I tried not to tighten my grip on Mother's hand, but it was the only sensation I could register that wasn't Greek Week in my ribcage. Involuntary, I managed to snort out a protest against waiting. If there was something burrowing its way through my intestines, time seemed to be a precious entitlement.

"I have some in my purse."

Mother, always prepared, pried her hand out of mine and scurried over to the other side of the room for her black leather bag. As she rummaged through the tissues and Tylenols, Wyndham stopped her.

"You can't do that! It has to go through our Pharmacy."

Mother looked over at me, helpless, visibly put off by the roadblock technicality. I, however, was now furious, and in defense mode from the grueling work out with which Wyndham was smashing the corners of my body. The pain, worse than ever now, jolted me to an up-right position in full on exorcist mode.

"FUCK YOU! FUCKING GIVE IT TO ME AND FUCK YOU!"

Gagging out words through the full body contractions, Mother came back across the room with a single, pink, dissolving tablet of anti-gas medication and popped it into my mouth. My hands were still glued to the broken sides of the bed, pulling ferociously at the rails to stabilize myself, searching for a position that would change, or dissipate the pain. Mother's hand found its way back into mine, perhaps hoping to sustain contact with me should I slip away. I continued to clamp down, continuing to sweat, and swear, and squeeze, and hope for a change. What the fuck was happening? Waiting for this thing, whatever it was, to just bore its way out of me already, I assumed through the broken blood vessels on my face, that this was, maybe, what childbirth felt like, if babies were born out of your liver. Make it stop!

Not five minutes later, still firmly attached to Mother's hand and the bedrail, the contractions and contortions of my insides subsided.

Class dismissed.

There was stillness in the room, a quiet. I was sore. Sore from the contractions, from the failed Morphine drip. Nurse Wyndham slowly inhaled and exhaled across the floor as she scurried out calling for CT scans and MRI's.

Two scans in the tubes of claustrophobia, and four hours later it turns out that the class was nothing but a blockage of gas and colitis. Good God, who knew that a little air could do that to a person? Completely worn out, unable, or unwilling to do anything I watched Nurse Wyndham hang the prep chemo on my IV bag. Mother and I sat peacefully, hand in hand, watching the Tony Awards as the clear poison slowly lurked its way back into my body.

Edward Miskie

223 Why, God?

Listening to Mother talk me into leaving, tucked under my comforter with a liter jug of water under my arm, and a thermometer held under my tongue, I starred at the wall and the sign I had made for myself.

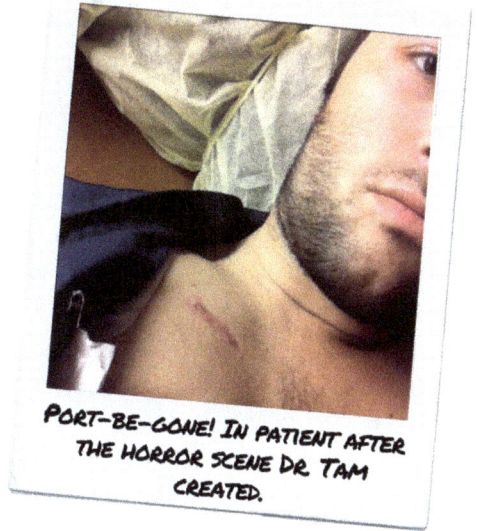

PORT-BE-GONE! IN PATIENT AFTER THE HORROR SCENE DR. TAM CREATED.

"Eat. Laugh. Leave."

It was my reminder that I had things to do even on days when I felt like staying in bed all day.

Eat something, even if I wasn't hungry or felt on the verge of vomit.

Laugh at something, anything, for any reason.

Leave the apartment, even if it was just a walk around the block or to the Starbucks on 168th Street for food I wasn't supposed to eat; two birds with one stone, as they say.

But now, freezing as I sweat under a comforter in the middle of June, I didn't want to do any of those things. All I wanted was to lie there and magically feel better; no doctors, no hospitals, no lengthy antibiotic drips or blood transfusions, just feel better.

The thermometer beeped.

"102.4."

Mother, in her soft-spoken kind of way, strongly suggested, short of demanded, that I get my things together and head East.

I called my roommate, Thuy, into my room to help me pack a bag and get a cab. Laptop, phone charger, water bottle, change of clothes, teddy bear. I gathered what strength I had and threw the seven-hundred-pound comforter off my fever-soaked body. I could barely sit or stand. Thuy appeared in the doorway and walked over to the bed, grabbing both of my arms and pulling me towards him, heaving me upwards. He took my arm, linking his through the crook of my elbow, grabbed my bag, and walked me to the corner of 163rd and Broadway.

I fell into the backseat of the taxi and decided to call the Emergency Room regarding my arrival. As the cab sped down through Harlem and the FDR Highway, I held myself up on my left elbow with my phone in my right hand pressed against my over-heated face.

"Hey guys, I'm on my way right now and I can't really walk; could someone please meet me at the entrance with a wheelchair?"

I was promised a wheelchair, but once I got there, freezing in the sweltering heat, there wasn't a chair or a soul around. Sliding out of the cab nearly face-planting on the sidewalk, I manipulated myself up onto two feet and stumbled my way through the fever haze into the annex. I supported what was left of me on the walls as I walked down the never-ending corridor, bouncing my body from wall to cubical partition, to wall until I had pin-balled my way to the Emergency Room entrance.

Two nurses, both more beautiful than the next, from what I could make out, sat at the big wooden desk in matching black. Nurse Yvonne handed me a clipboard with a stack of papers on it while Nurse Yvette gave instructions.

"Fill those out please."

A bead of sweat slid down the bridge of my nose and landed smack dab in the middle of the information sheets. The cloud that had fogged my vision was thickening, and focusing on anything, let alone tiny print on white pages, was increasingly getting more difficult, scary. All of my weight was on the top of the desk. My legs had all but fallen out from underneath me. My knees buckled against the front of the desk relying on my upper body and grip on the clipboard and pen to support it from slinking to the floor.

"I'm sorry, but I don't think I have time for that. I'm going down."

Nurse Yvonne assured me I'd be fine and gestured me to the seating area behind me that somehow, I had missed. Stumbling into one of the leather chairs I adjusted myself in a way that I could hold my body up. I had reached a point where I couldn't do it on my own. I signed some papers. I checked my fever.

The shade of my skin was beginning to fade from a healthy-ish tan to flush white and chalky. All the pigment was visually evacuating my body. Not even my melanin wanted to be a part of this anymore. I wondered if this is what dying felt like; clammy, heavy, and hot.

Nurse Kim walked out of the triage room and half carried me into a mini side-room off the waiting area to take my vitals. One hundred and two point four had climbed to a staggering one hundred and four. Strongly appealing to Nurse Kim to please give me a goddamn gurney to, at the very least, lie down and die on so as to not have to resort to the floor, she agreed. I was taken into the back of the Emergency Room check in area, and placed in a cordoned off curtain cubicle, in a bed.

Lying there, barely moving, slipping in and out of consciousness, surrounded by blue curtains, sweating and shaking, waiting and worrying, I called Father. The sound of Father's phone ringing in my ear persisted as Nurse Kim swooped in past the partitions like a chopper. In her hand was a box of blood vials.

"Could I get some water please? I really feel like I need water."

No water. No saline. No fluids until blood was drawn, and the source of the fever was determined. Not even a glass of water. A change of sheets would have been nice, seeing as I had soaked them from merely laying there having blood extracted. Three vials in, Father picked up the phone with predetermined worry in his voice. Mother must have told him of the high fever and my intent to make way to Sloan.

"You should get here. I'm worried. It's not good. Please!"

He hung up and booked the next Amtrak to The City, as he and Mother often did. Nurse Kim swooped up the box of blood vials and assured me that fluids were on the way.

"May I at least pee? I have to go to the bathroom!"

She returned in a few moments with a wheelchair. Better late than never. Monkey-barring from the bed to the chair, I plopped down onto the seat nearly breaking apart entirely. Nurse Kim, nearly the same size as the wheelchair, slowly pushed me across the room to the single-person lavatory.

My frail, rickety body made its way out of the chair and slid along the wall into the bathroom. Behind the locked door, I braced myself wall to wall, grasping onto the texture of the wallpaper as my only traction to stay upright. I took a deep breath, making sure I was steady and ready. Coffee came out. What looked like weak, sad coffee that I would never even consider drinking, was releasing from my body. Hot, brown sludge furiously shot into the clear water of the bowl splattering Pollock dots onto the walls and sides of the basin. My eyes locked in terror on the hue that was taking over the porcelain. I had seen this once in a movie starring Phillip Seymour Hoffman in which he was living a life but was actually a dead person. Was I about to be a dead person?

Fuck.

Pumping the antiseptic lotion dispenser on the wall, I lathered my mortality around in the palms of my hands. What the actual fuck was going on inside me? Nurse Kim got me back across the room to my cage where an IV pole of saline fluids was awaiting my return. No need to tell her about the French press, then. Sleep, rest, and peace all came upon me long enough that when I awoke, Father was sitting in a chair inside the emergency room curtain-cage waiting for me to wake up.

"You have a staph infection in your port that has moved into your blood."

Fantastic! Father gathered my things and followed Nurse Kim to the fifth floor, the Urology floor, the only floor where there was room to put me. Evidently cancer was afoot.

I remained in bed, unable to move much, for four days. Once the antibiotic juggling-act was complete, I found myself shirtless in my hospital bed, under a sterile pad, and Dr. Tam. There were no signs of pomp and circumstance that one would anticipate under surgical expectations, just Dr. Tam and his henchmen Dr. Thomas in my hospital room, there to remove my port. Like being backed up against the wall, I was informed of the ports removal as they sterilized the right side of my chest with brown, stinging solution. The starchy sheets were pulled up to my abdomen for me. The operating instruments rested on my stomach. The team began to dig.

Father was on the other side of the room clear in my line of vision, literally backed up against the wall. I could see flashes of his worried face, periodically obstructed by Dr. Tam's hand guiding the knife across my chest. Unable to see anything else, I watched Father's flushed face sheepishly watch the scalpel's drag, trying not to look, but unable to look away.

Like a bow that was gliding across the bridge of a cello, back and forth the scalpel went, slowly cutting me open, playing me like a fiddle. Soon the scalpel was replaced with a large pair of scissors, that looked more so as if they were designed to cut cardboard, and nothing that would have been lodged in a body.

Dr. Tam inserted the scissors into the hole he created in my chest and began to cut, as if I were a product inside a meat counter. Chicken cutlets? Father looked increasingly disturbed in his silence, only jolted by the clap of the scissors or the thick garbled instructions infrequently garbling out of Dr. Tam thin lips.

"One more cut."

Seizing open and shut on the final piece, it felt as though we'd struck steel, stone, or bone. Dr. Tam's grip graduated to a two-hander, squeezing the scissors inward and inward, shaking the apparatus out of my body and back in. My body began to rock up and down with each push and squeeze, and the calm of trust began to fade.

"Damn it! It's calcified. Damn it!"

Dr. Thomas placed his hand on my right shoulder as Dr. Tam continued to wrestle with the encrypted port, clapping the scissors blades together, violently trying to set it free. Bouncing up and down, I felt as though my insides were going to bounce out of the hole in my chest with the ferocity that Dr. Tam was trying to cut into this entombed deposit. I was just about to reach for the guardrails on the side of the bed to stabilize my rocking chair-like CPR convulsions, when a fan of red shot from my chest. It was blood, a short spray of blood. Like a lawn sprinkler it spattered the ceiling, the wall, the bed, the ceiling, Dr. Tam's un-masked, un-goggled face, and me.

I began to laugh uncontrollably, as Dr. Tam stitched the opening up.

"Hold still!"

Oh, now you want me to hold still! Part of my hysterics was the visual of the horror movie blood spray, part of it was the fact that I could relax a little and knowing the absence of that very port meant that I'd get to live another day.

Edward Miskie

224 Man in Chair

I sat in the middle of the empty room staring at the medical posters of cross-section human diagrams tacked onto the wall, and the empty exam chairs below them. Exam chairs exactly like the one that I was confined to; wide, beige, upholstered in cheap pleather with two arm rests. It was Stem Cell collection time again, and I was getting antsy from the immobile itinerary Sloan Kettering had laid out for me. They had kept me inpatient

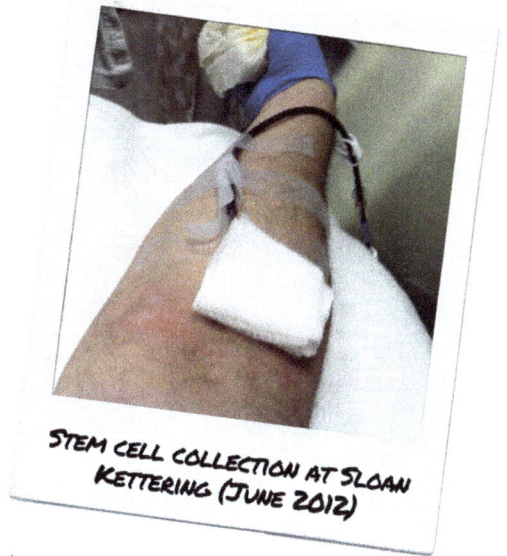

STEM CELL COLLECTION AT SLOAN KETTERING (JUNE 2012)

from my infected port fiasco, as the timing was convenient to begin collection. Now ten days on the inside, I was getting antsy. I wasn't allowed to walk down to my collection appointments; it was hospital policy that I was wheeled down in a wheelchair, or gurney. There were no creepy prison GPS tracking devices at Sloan. So, all I did, all I could do, was sit in my chair, stare at the wall, and listen to Musical Theatre.

Trying to look past my stagnant seated confinement, I tried to remain chipper and upbeat. This was my second attempt at collecting Stem Cells, and even though the first time at Manhattan County Hospital didn't go very well, this time, I was having collection done right. There was no Bactrim in my system inhibiting my Stem Cells from generating, there were a few months of recoup time behind me, and I was at a hospital I trusted with my life - literally. And though, in all regards, I was in upgrade territory, the surroundings, the sound of the machine, Mother sitting at my side reading a magazine, all snapped me back into the last time I had done this whole sitting-in-a-chair-going-nowhere thing four months before.

Before the breakup, Valentine came to The City for Valentine's Day.

With a two-inch metal needle in my arm, that looked more like a Bic pen then a medical instrument, I sat, trapped, in a reclining chair connected to a machine. It was my first day of Stem Cell collection at Manhattan County Hospital and, unable to move, the hours were ticking by painfully slowly. Valentine was on one side of me, attached to his phone as usual, and on the other side was a gay couple, likely in their seventies, holding hands. One of them was also hooked up to a similar machine as I was.

It was daunting, touching, but daunting. Was this my future? With such love and commitment to a person, a person in their worst form, the worst circumstances you would imagine, still holding hands and resting one's head on the other's shoulder, I managed to look past the cancer, and the hospital, and smiled at them.

"I don't like that picture at all."

My head snapped left to right, furrowing my brow at Valentine's statement. His face was buried in his phone, still, shifting view from our game of Hanging with Friends to the older couple. I wasn't sure if he meant the cancer part, or the growing old part, but nearly a second after he said it, the familiar chime of a 'social app' went off. We both ignored it.

Thankfully, I didn't have to worry about Mother cruising 'social apps' while I sat in the familiar chair, but the same Bic pen was in my arm, and I was still stuck in a chair unable to go anywhere, still willing Stem Cells to be produced. And I had my Broadway! Every few songs, I'd pull out an earbud and relay to Mother what I was listening to and why it was so brilliant, but still I was strapped into the dialysis machine, unable to go anywhere.

At least lunch was provided. And by lunch on the third day of collection, veins in my left forearm having turned hard and tendon-like, I was begging Nurse Trix to let me eat outside. All I wanted was to get up, walk around, and feel the outside. After four hours of cheeky begging had turned into frustrated demands, Nurse Trix, with a wink and a smile, came along and unhooked me from the stationary airplane seat of an exam chair. She let me stumble along the hallway to the outside, setting me free into the afternoon.

"Don't leave the sidewalk in front of the door. I'll be watching."

Unhooked, with my boxed hospital lunch, Mother led me through reception to the front doors.

"Are you sure you want to go outside?"

After days of being confined to a chair?

"ARE YOU KIDDING?"

With gusto, I grabbed the black bar on the door, and slammed it open exposing the outside. The hot June air was almost too thick to inhale, but the embrace of it was comforting, contrasting against my body that was, now, familiar only to central air. The fanfare of traffic and pedestrians swelled through the now open door like an overture. Newspapers, and abandoned leaves, the only real nature in The City, kicked up in the breeze. The businessmen, and women of the Upper East Sixties danced, and pivoted around each other, like a movie-set from the days of MGM. As they passed, they smiled at me, breaking into fan kicks and double turns. Even the newsstand attendee seemed to be singing with the honk and speed of the pedestrians and taxis.

Standing on the sidewalk to the left of the main entrance, fighting the urge not to join the choreography of First Avenue, I nibbled on the tiny tuna sandwich as slowly as possible so as to not cut my sweet, glorious freedom short. I tilted my head back as I chewed, facing the trees lining the avenue with my arms gently outstretched at my sides. I closed my eyes taking in the loveliness that was the outdoors. Halal cart deliciousness replaced the smell of The City (urine and money), and nostalgia crept in from years ago when I was living off street-meat and Jamba Juice, and unable to hold a job for long. All of that seemed so far away, lifetimes ago. If only the Cancer version of me could tell the disaster version of me what was coming.

I dusted the crumbs of the tuna sandwich off my hospital gown, I took in a heavy breath, and let out a weighty sigh, savoring the fresh-ish air of The City.

"Ready to go back in?"

I hugged Mother. The passers-by seemed to have stopped their zealous commute. The newsstand attendee was simply handing out change to the disgruntled doctors, and administrators. Traffic had moved on, and it seemed, it was time for me to do so as well.

"No!"

Mother laughed. We both turned to go back inside where Nurse Trix was waiting at the front desk, watching me, waiting for me to come back in, making sure I wasn't going to make a break for it.

On the last day of vacuuming my blood stream of Stem Cells, I sat silent, no musical theatre, no demands for the outside. Dr. Anthony informed me that I had barely collected enough Stem Cells to do the transplant, including the few that we carted over from my previous medical residence. I was disappointed in myself. With the metal spear in my arm, I remained still throughout the last appointment, convinced that speaking was too much of a strain on the Stem Cells; they wouldn't come out of me if I exerted myself too much. So, my mouth remained shut, and my phone remained silent. I just sat there staring at my phone conscious of my every move, wary of my body's overachieving in the underachieving department.

I was officially out of 'tomorrow will be betters.' And as Nurse Trix pulled the metal needle out of me for the final time, a warm feeling of accepting my helplessness and fate traveled with me in the wheelchair back to my room. Freedom from this invisible looming fetter seemed dimmer than it had before, and what hope I had left was shaky at best. I began to return to the hole I hadn't fallen into for quite some time.

Back in my hospital room, reclined in another chair, I waited for Dr. Anthony and the official word, the final collection results. Did we have enough? Had I psyched myself up for no reason? Was I going to have to do the Allogenic Transplant after all? Fuck! What was going to happen to me? Fate contemplations were abruptly interrupted with the entrance of Dr. Anthony bursting through the door with a tall, bespectacled, respectable looking man that the very sight of, brought my leather chair to an upright position.

"This is Dr. Gloriosus; he will be head of your transplant team."

Praise the lord and saints alive there is a God. If this was going to be the head of my transplant team, I was going to really love this transplant. Ok, like, not really actually love it, but at least have something to push me through it other than leaving.

As Dr. Anthony spoke, I only half registered what she was saying, which may, or may not have included information about the number of Stem Cells I collected. Which may or may not have included information about the number of Stem Cells I had not collected. We were at bare bones minimum. WONDERFUL! I didn't even mind. The man whose hands my life was in was the exact replica of every hot, laboratory, stud-nerd you've ever seen. His sunken bright eyes, behind his Warby Parker's, and the disheveled dirty-blond, wavy hair that sat, tousled atop his head. His white lab coat, and perfectly tied tie were like a daydream. His charcoal dress pants, and recently shined Allen Edmonds burrowed themselves into my memory. He didn't have scrubs on, so I knew he was important.

He exuded this shy arrogance that could only convey that he knew exactly what the fuck he was doing, and he was going to fuck up my cancer, and I couldn't fucking wait. And even though I was still shitting-my-pants scared of 'bringing you to the brinks of death with chemo and revive you with stem cells,' if this hot-doc was going to be heading the project, then let the fucking games begin!

Edward Miskie

23 I'm Calm

Senex, being a former Marine, gave me a run for my money as we sped around the racetrack the seventh floor at Sloan Kettering had become. Sliding around the corners on my socks, or on the wheels of the IV pole past those already in isolation; a direction I was inevitably headed, we made the most of my stay. There was a refreshment center in the middle of the stretch of hall around the corner from my room filled with coffee, tea, and juices.

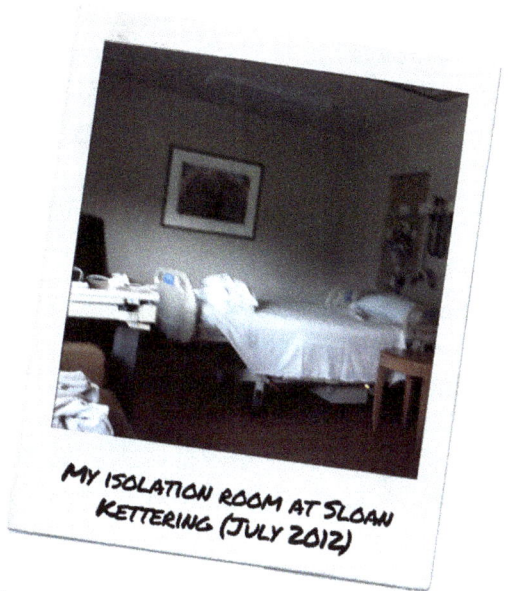

MY ISOLATION ROOM AT SLOAN KETTERING (JULY 2012)

Fourteen laps in, Senex and I decided to stop for a drive-by apple juice.

Inside the refreshment alcove was another man, about my age, maybe a little older, in a similar hospital gown as mine, with a similar haircut to mine, bald, pouring a cup of tea. He introduced himself as Hero.

"So, what are you in for?"

Apparently, I had turned into a sitcom from the hospital oxygen I was huffing from all the laps around the floor. Lightening the mood was not on this guy's radar, which was completely understandable, because cancer is a horseshit wave to be riding, but as I picked out an apple juice from the fridge, excusing my IV pole in the tight space, he murmured back to me through the yellow facemask looped around his ears.

"Leukemia."

Senex and I both stood there watching him stir his tea following the motion of the tinted water and stirring straw.

"They told me to stay away from germs; I have three young kids. How am I supposed to do that and be a dad?"

149

Suddenly my problems and circumstance didn't seem so bad. If I died, I didn't have kids to leave behind, but I still had the $1,200 I'd saved from avoiding having them. Senex and I made a path for Hero to pass through, and my two cents found its way in a place where it didn't belong.

"You can't be a dad to them now so you can be a dad to them later."

He turned around with his tea in his hand, his mask blocking most of any expression he may, or may not have made, but he just kind of, maybe, smiled and nodded his head before walking away back into his room. I need to learn to keep my mouth shut.

The final lap around the floor was a somber one, lacking the IV pole rides and sock skidding around the corners. Neither Senex nor I really said much after meeting Hero. As we approached the final few feet of the hallway, dragging my IV pole alongside, I stopped dead in my tracks grabbing Senex's arm. On the corner, the room next to mine with the big windows was empty.

"I want it!"

The beautiful Nurse Philia, with her long blond hair, and equally long legs, helped me move next-door. Together, the three of us carried extra pillows into the room to princess the place up, propping each pillow against the arm of the big, brown, leather sofa. I was definitely sleeping on the sofa. Despite hospital changes, the beds were still horrendously uncomfortable, like there's only one hospital bed provider in the whole industry, striving to make those in need of them miserable.

A subconscious tension I'd been holding on to since I arrived relaxed at the sight of my new digs. The lay out of the room was huge, rectangular, and had double the windows containing a view that didn't include a wall. And even though it was nighttime, if I kneeled on the sofa and leaned over the windowsill, I could see a partial view of Rockefeller University and The Caspary Auditorium. Trees! I decided that I was going to like it in this new room, as much as one can like being in a hospital, being inundated with chemo and their own bodily fluids to save their life. Senex offered to spend the night to make sure I was going to be ok. I was going to be ok, but I accepted his offer as to avoid being alone.

The sun beat through the window the following morning, my blanket hugging my shoulders, my teddy bear nestled in the crook of my arm, and Senex sitting at the desk with coffee.

"They woke me up last night for vitals. They thought I was you."

Mother walked through the door to the two of us chuckling over the late-night mix-up. She was alarmed, unaware that we had changed rooms, thinking something horrendous had happened without her being notified. Mother gave me a hug, handed me a coffee, and took Senex's seat at the desk as he headed out into July to get his day started.

Mother opened her bag and shuffled through some papers in her tote, pulling out a stack of documents resembling a cement block. There were so many papers. She placed the pages on the hospital bed while I sipped my coffee and pried open my laptop to continue where I had left off on my last ThereAreGiants article.

Mother's frittering over her vast file cabinet of paperwork distracted my focus of vision from my computer screen to her. She was standing over the hospital bed, the piles of paperwork all categorized and stacked by date. The way she was ticking away, silently mapping out the past eight months of medical mail was nothing short of awe-inspiring meticulousness. I watched her seal each categorized mountain of bills, correspondence, and notices in their assigned giant zip-lock freezer bags. I hadn't noticed until this exact moment, but that's where I got it. That's where I got my obsessive, organizing, weird, alphabetized, sizing, crazy. Evidently, I was a lot more like my mother than I had previously been aware. I had always thought I was more like my father, which is not incorrect, but this moment hit me, watching Mother go ape shit on a stack of papers. Family!

Once all the freezer bags had been lined up like plastic file folders inside Mother's tote, she sat and picked up her phone to check messages from the family group-text. And then Dr. Gloriosus entered the room for his regular morning visit.

Dr. Gloriosus was my favorite part of the day. He was better than coffee. Even though he was typically delivering news that wasn't related to my leaving the hospital, not being allowed to take a shower because I was a falling hazard, the chemo was working so my immune system was crashing; he was my great escape for the two and a half minutes he stood in my doorway.

The door's swift opening created a breeze that tousled the doctor's hair high atop his Warby Parker's. His slow-motion gaze from the doorknob over to me, reclining on the sofa with his bedroom eyes, made my heart flutter, and my stomach hurt. He swung his clipboard into his line of vision, reviewing the numbers and results of my latest bloodwork for the chorus in training he led into the room behind him, and me. I barely noticed the chorus.

"By the looks of things, I think you're ready for your transplant. We will be in tomorrow to discuss moving forward."

Already? I looked over at Mother who was already examining the spreadsheet of blood counts she had been clocking since day one of the long haul. I guess it had been nine days of chemo, which was the projected protocol. Between editor meetings for ThereAreGiants, writing articles, and hospital room parties with friends, I had lost all track of time in the monotony of my daily lack of routine.

From other's accounts, I had expected a lot more gloom and doom from this experience. I was anticipating a lot more barfing, sprinting to the bathroom and not making it, hot flashes, lethargy, hustle to save my limp, lifeless body when the inevitable went wrong. Sure, I had lost some energy, weight, and hair, but overall, I didn't feel like complete death, but more so just weakened and bored; cautious. All was eerily calm. I didn't move too much, or force activity outside of my laps around the floor in hopes of avoiding more complications. The last thing I needed was a repeat of early June's ocean-parasite, eating my body from the inside out without any antibodies to fight it off, frantically hoping the nursing staff would inject me with more steroids, wondering if this was the end.

Breakfast arrived as Dr. Gloriosus listed some basic instructions and advice for the next twenty-four hours. Completely relying on Mother to take in his instructions, I tuned him out and looked at the meal I was about to force feed myself. Only food takes precedence over hot doctors. It was happening. Was this the end; a notion I pondered far too much in the span of eight months? I lifted the lid of the hot tray of food to the eggs and bacon I had ordered, subconsciously wondering if this was my last breakfast. I picked up a piece of bacon and put the meat in my mouth returning my attention back to the doctor.

"Your numbers have hit absolute zero. Until we tell you otherwise, you can't leave this room."

He turned his back on me, his white coat like a cape trailing behind him as he closed the door, leaving me staring out the window of the door, looking at the seventh floor.

Oh boy. Here we go.

24 Three Little Words

Four pizzas. All I wanted was four pizzas from the hospital kitchen for Anthony, Dionne, Claude, Senex, and I. Isolation was a drag, and in an effort to remain feeling normal for as long as I could, I threw a party in my room. Definitely the loudest room on the floor, we all sat around in gowns, masks, and gloves being a complete nuisance.

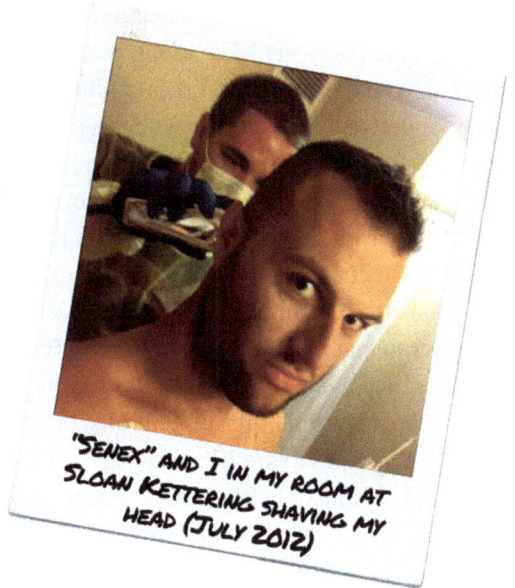

"SENEX" AND I IN MY ROOM AT SLOAN KETTERING SHAVING MY HEAD (JULY 2012)

"Shh! Guys, I can't hear!"

Everyone quieted down so I could place the order for the pizza party. I felt like a soccer mom whose turn it was to feed the kids cheap take-out after the game.

"You're only permitted one meal per order."

Rain. Parade. I looked around the room at each of my friends, suffocating behind the unpleasant, itchy, hot masks with assuredness instilled in me that I knew who my friends were. I would do anything for any one of these people, including throwing a bitch fit at the hospital kitchen for pizzas.

"Ok, well I'd really love four pizzas just this once if that's ok?"

No. It was not ok and sending my friends out into the sweltering twilight heat felt cruel when air-conditioning and food was available right where we were. Also, I couldn't leave, and I was lonely and needy for warm bodies to be in the same room as me. I was not sending them away.

I promised myself that I wouldn't do this, it felt so gross and disgusting, and before I even said it, I hated myself, but I wanted fucking pizza.

"So, I'm like having a transplant here and may not actually leave this hospital alive, so can I please just get four fucking pizzas?"

The second I said it I regretted it. I swore I'd never use the Cancer Card ever again, and not only did I just use it, but I used it like a basic bitch, in my own hospital, with the staff that was providing me food. The sinking feeling of disappointment and assholedness descended through the end of my hand into the phones cradle as I hung up with the food service line. Only Dionne gave me the side eye before continuing with our Stem Cell Transplant pizza party. Though I remained outwardly conversational with my friends, I couldn't shake the familiar feeling I had curated back in December, at the very beginning of cancer.

Manhattan County Hospital was expecting me any day now and I began to surrender to that idea, so I drank. I drank Bulleit Rye in a glass tumbler with three ice cubes, and a lengthy order of Sushi from Seamless that kept me company. Somewhere between Philadelphia rolls, bourbon, and checking Seymour's size every five minutes to see if he had shrunk, hoping all of this would go away, I worked myself up to believe that the second I started chemo I was going to lose every hair I ever grew. No one had told me otherwise, except one doctor who mentioned during a demonstration of wigs for men that some people don't lose their hair at all. Knowing my luck, I had gotten cancer after all, I'd be bald within twenty seconds of the starting line and sitting in a pile of my own follicles. Near next to panicked, with a side of dread at the idea of heading downtown, I decided to make a pilgrimage to the H&M in midtown to stock up on stylish hats in an effort to counter what was about to happen.

I exited the subway station and tried to turn the corner where I was met with an extraordinarily large crowd of tourists that had all converged-on Rockefeller Center for the goddamn Christmas Tree lighting. This is one of the worst cluster-fucks in New York City events. Sure, it's pretty, and maybe you consider it to be 'a thing' that one should do, but similar to anything else where streets are blocked off and vehicular and foot traffic are obstructed, it's one of those special Hells that only New Yorkers truly experience and avoid. Here I was in the middle of it all ambling up Sixth Avenue, caged in by the official New York Police Department cattle shoots used to herd the crowds during such events. I moved with the crowd trying to find a way over to Fifth Avenue to continue on my hat quest.

Officer Oda Mae instructed me to walk up Sixth Avenue on the western side of the block to Fifty Fourth Street and cross. I did, but then wasn't able to get to Fifth Avenue from the other side of Sixth.

"You in danger, girl!"

Tell me about it. Between cancer, and these crowds, I was basically scared for my life.

Around and around, I went until I finally got to Fifth avenue; the wrong side of Fifth Avenue opposite of where H&M sits. Pissed, and blockaded from crossing the street, staring directly at H&M with only a waist high metal grate and a cluster of cops in my way, I was over it. I was not about to walk in circles for another forty-five minutes for a ten-dollar hat, so I approached the gaggle of policemen standing on the favorable side of the barricades.

"Hey. Could you guys please let me cross? I'm just trying to get to H&M."

Of course, The Heat who decided to take on this sweaty disgruntled nuisance just happened to be the tallest and hunkiest of the bunch with his tossed hair, cleft chin, perfect teeth, square jaw, and bulging arms. Officer Sam Wheat.

"Sorry, buddy, you have to walk up to 54th Street and..."

UGH!

"Yeah, I just did all of that and here I am... on this side of the street."

Officer Wheat didn't budge.

"Sorry, buddy, that's the traffic pattern for the tree lighting. You gotta walk up to 54th Street to cross and then make your way..."

The enchantment in his cleft chin and arms began to fade under my frustrations. I no longer cared that he looked like a Greek statue stuffed into a policeman's uniform that might as well have been partially painted on. I just wanted a hat, and my bed, and my bourbon, and I began to lose it.

"OFFICER! I don't give a fucking shit about the goddamn tree lighting. I am starting chemo this week, and all my hair is going to fall out, and all I want to do is cross the fucking street to buy a fucking hat at the fucking H&M that is RIGHT OVER THERE! I! HAVE! CANCER!"

The second the words came out of my mouth I felt it begin to fold up like a Venus Fly Trap. I shut up. The crazy spilled all over this uniformed fantasy and my body restarted shaking, humming. That nervous jitter you get when you're auditioning, or are about to get on a big, fast amusement park ride. My insides were buzzing, and no matter how hard I tried to still myself, or fight off the single Evan Rachel Wood tear, I wasn't budging. Officer Wheat sighed, looking directly at me. God, he was good looking.

"Alright. Come with me."

His imposing hands lifted up the metal barrier like it was paper and pulled it towards his thick thighs. His colleagues were looking at me with a nauseating combination of pity and concern. I walked through the channel he opened for me following him across Fifth Avenue. His silence was arousing. He very gently, and almost apologetically, lifted the cages on the other side of the street.

"Thank you!"

Two steps towards the front door, Wheat chopped into my pace.

"Good luck."

I stopped in my tracks and turned to face his painful-to-look-at handsome mug. Good luck? Finding a hat?

"Yeah, Fuck you."

Gliding up the escalator in the middle of the massive store, it occurred to me that I'd played the Cancer Card for the first time, and I played it hard! Did I feel good about this? Playing up a horrible disadvantage to get something that I wanted that I couldn't have gotten otherwise: this should have tickled me, right? Get what you can from a crap circumstance, right? I repeated the three little words to myself again as I made my way through the overflowing racks of clothes.

"I have cancer."

Nope! I definitely didn't like the sound of that.

Sifting through the few hat choices, I selected the options that I liked, and tried them on. I looked at myself in the mirror, concentrating, trying to picture myself bald, hiding my hair under the seams of the hats. There were two faux fur lined trapper hats and two knitted skullcaps. I got all four. The fur ones hid the shape of my head and any trace of where hair would have been. The skullcaps were a little too real for me, but, hey, for ten dollars? Fine!

The cashier checked out my purchase and placed the receipt in the bag. I kept replaying Officer Wheat's good luck wishes. Good luck finding a fucking hat. What a dick! As if finding a hat was difficult, or something I wasn't capable of doing; fuck him and his perfect genetics. I grabbed my shopping bag, thanking the cashier, and turned to rush out of the store back into the nightmare tree lighting crowds. From the front door of the store, across the street, remained the NYPD. Their backs were turned, probably discussing what a spectacle I made. So embarrassing. I supposed in hindsight a cop being a snarky dick about finding a hat wasn't a battle I should fight in my head compared to the scheduled battle I had on deck.

I looked down at the shopping bag. Mission accomplished. Time to go home. As I walked back towards the train, looking behind me at the NYPD, I said it to myself one more time trying to bring myself to a reality of the concept.

"I have Cancer."

And with a sick, sinking feeling from my forehead down, I realized, not ten steps down the street, he didn't mean good luck finding a stupid hat.

The pizza arrived. I got what I wanted. I ate the pizza, but I felt like shit doing so.

Edward Miskie

24.1 Regretful-Happy

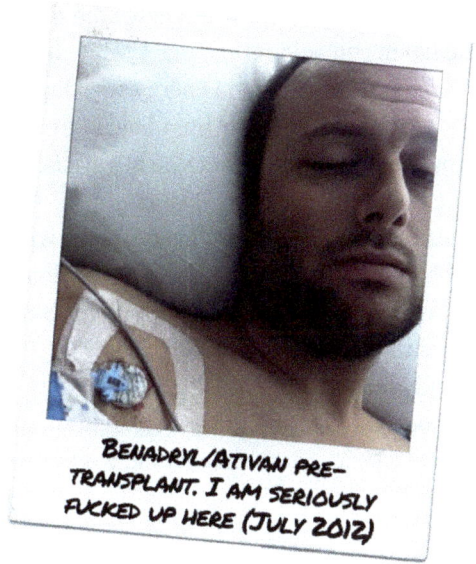

BENADRYL/ATIVAN PRE-TRANSPLANT. I AM SERIOUSLY FUCKED UP HERE (JULY 2012)

"Let's fucking do this shit!"

The Benadryl and Ativan cocktail drip had set in, and I was writhing under the sheets of the hospital bed I had now, finally, been forced into. The figures in the room were still and backlit from the sun pouring in through the big windows. Dark outlines of Dr. Anthony, Dr. Gloriosus, and Mother loomed at the foot and sides of the bed like an episode of the X-Files. I wasn't ready for this. I was supposed to have a day of rest between my last day of chemo and the actual Stem Cell infusion. I had planned on using that day to mentally prepare for this, but for whatever reason, be it time or circumstance, we dove straight into the infusion: no day of rest, no mental preparation.

A shadow approached my IV pole which had been stripped of the decorations from friends that hung on it to brighten the mood of room. The shadow lifted a balloon-like bag and hung it on one of the metal rings high atop the chemo tree. It was the infusion, my Stem Cells, a bag full of my fluids. It was big, and swollen, and a nauseating shade of red. Something about it reminded me of raw ground beef thrown into a blender and put in water.

During my medicated swim in the sheets, and the bags of downers emptying into my veins, I began to let go of whatever was going to happen next. It was too late. It was too late to change my mind. It was too late to stop. As the Benadryl clouds grew thicker, and my consciousness grew thin, hearing only the countdown of the infusions start coming from a warped, husky voice, I let go and slipped into uncharted quiet waters, not knowing if I'd come back.

Startled and awake, I found myself scrunched up on the leather bed-couch clinging to my ratty, old teddy bear wondering how I got there. The last thing I remembered was going under for the second time, for the second half of the Stem Cell infusion. The preservatives in the Stem Cells were already making me nauseous, faster and in a way that chemo never had, even having been awake for only a few minutes. It was a new kind of sick, a new kind of discourse inside me, like having an acid reflux attack while being severely hung over.

All my attention and energy was directed at my digestive track and my refusal to allow myself to throw up. I hated throwing up. I don't think people liking throwing up is a thing, but you always hear of some creepo who's into getting puked on, so who knows. No judgment. All I knew is that the few-and-far between times I had misplaced my insides were wildly unpleasant.

Now firing on all cylinders, I was doing everything I could to aggressively suppress what was decidedly going to come out of me, one way or another. Mother was sitting quietly in her chair, unaware of the lid I was trying to hold down, and literally hold down what little I had ingested in the last two days. The tenseness of my body choking my teddy bear in my frail forearms loosened after a few strategic attempts at Zen, nasal-inhalation, meditative wishing, but eventually, I gave up.

"Mother, I'm going to be sick."

She didn't even look at me before springing out of the chair across the room and diving into the bathroom. Frisbee throwing a mauve color basin onto the floor just beneath my head, it barely landed in time for me to roll over and contract, orally giving birth to a hunter green ocean. Mother began frantically pressing the nurses call button for help as The Hoover Dam continued to fill the basin to the brim. There was no way that this color, this volume, and this frequency was normal. I was dying. I was definitely dying. With each heave, I began to run the checklist of funeral preferences I had specified in my head, as Nurse Phila entered the room.

"Oh, that's totally normal. The mucous membrane lining of your entire body is being rejected, leaving the body to re-line itself. You're fine."

Totally normal is not how I would have described that event at all, but now, without an internal lining, shit was real. Nurse Philia let us know, as she left the room, that I was 'there,' I was standing on very fragile ground. As calmly as she entered, having emptied the basin in the toilet, she disappeared back into the now foreign seventh floor.

Like nothing had happened, Mother and I sat in silence punching out sentences on our respective devices in the hermetically sealed room, shaken by the alien occurrences in the basin. The updated chart that Mother had been tracking my blood counts on had taken a numerical dip below zero. Four days into not leaving my room, I had a lot of time to get into my head about the next few days to come, weeks, if I even had that long.

The silence had gotten the better of Mother.

"Eddie."

She always called me Eddie. Only family is allowed to call me Eddie, but the tone of inquisitiveness was different. It was shaky, maybe timid. Mother isn't even remotely as boisterous as the rest of the family, but this was a little sheepish, even for her.

"Do you have any regrets?"

She tiptoed through the question. What? What was she talking about? Regrets like, I wish I hadn't finished that bottle of bourbon? I wish I hadn't hooked up with that guy. I wish I hadn't eaten my way through my early twenties? What regrets?

"Anything in your childhood you would change?"

And with that sentence, that question, it occurred to me: Mother was worried. There had been so many chances throughout the last eight months, this whole ordeal, to ask me anything she wanted. I mean, we had been talking about shit, puke, and sperm at every turn of treatment, so anything else that she may have wanted to know would likely be a thin wager against past topics of conversation. But now, sitting through the Les Misérables of treatment protocol, it seemed the severity and reality of the circumstances had gotten the better of her. Maybe, if it had gotten the better of her, perhaps I should be slightly more concerned than I had numbed myself to be.

Regrets. This felt like deathbed confessions. I put my laptop aside on the floor and hugged my knees into my chest, sifting through memories, sifting through possibilities I could potentially add to the tally of what Mother was asking.

One thing did come to mind.

A.I.M. opened up on the desktop of the family computer as I adjusted my comfort level in the overused computer chair. The chat windows of friends wondering what I was doing on this Friday night made a small stack on the main screen, but too late. I had just gotten home from seeing "Love Actually" and I had homework to do. I was a sophomore in high school and should, maybe, dedicate some time to schoolwork. As I closed the few messages out, one, stuck on the bottom of the stack, stuck out.

"I know you knew him. Read this."

The fist of the news punched me in the throat. My eyes were on fire as I read the notice from the college where I secretly attended LGBT meetings. That's where I had met him. That's where I met Robert Darling. When I told my parents I was going to a friend's house or coffee shop with others, that's really where I was going. That's where I could be myself. Nothing ever turned physical, but our conversations were rousing for a sixteen-year-old closeted gay boy; like discovering a new land. But he was gone. Gone?

Leaving the chat window open without responding, I ran into the kitchen and threw up in the sink. Mother and Father, taken aback, asked if I was ok. They knew about him, but not really, or how, or why, but having not been out to them just yet, I explained the abridged, safe version.

"He was killed in a car accident this afternoon."

My only thought, through my disbelief, was to call my tenth-grade religion teacher, Mrs. Amy. Her daughter, Sarah and I were friends, so I convinced myself there was trust enough to speak with her regarding such a matter as death. Despite the late hour, I began frantically dialing her home phone number from outside on to the back patio, hoping not to wake my sisters. The phone began to ring, and with each passing tone I could feel myself boiling from the inside.

"Hello?"

She sounded confused by the late call and the hysterics that came blaring through the phone receiver.

"Ed? I can't understand a thing you're saying. Why don't you come over for lunch tomorrow and we can talk? Are you going to be okay?"

Numb is the same as okay, right? I went to bed, but so many thoughts were whizzing through my brain. I could barely quiet myself down enough to close my eyes longer than five minutes. I think I regretted calling Mrs. Amy. What had I started? It was a long night. And when the sun did finally come up, I could barely bring myself to step out of bed. A sense of regret came over me, barely recalling my last conversation with the newly deceased. I had taken him for granted. Of course, he'd always be there to talk to. But he wouldn't. He'd never get out of bed again so why should I? Taking a shower felt wrong. Getting dressed felt rude. Everything I was doing was laden with the reminder that whatever I was doing, he was never going to do again.

Driving over to Mrs. Amy's home I felt blank; uncertain of even what to say to her or what about. How was I going to approach this? Was I really about to come out to my pious religion teacher? No. I definitely did not want to do that. I started to regret this approach and eased up on the gas pedal. How I was even going to speak to her about this got murkier, and muddier the closer I got to her house, until I found myself sitting in her driveway in my green Chrysler Cirrus. My car keys were in my hand. Mrs. Amy was standing in the doorway staring at me. I needed to talk to someone. This must have been it.

She hugged me in the threshold of the side door of her house leading me inside to the kitchen table. Maybe this wasn't going to be so bad. I sat in front of the salad and struck up small talk that I knew and felt was quickly tapering off. She was planted in her chair, fork in hand peering at me over her thick-rimmed glasses, almost waiting for the ribbon of bullshit to pull at its finish. I didn't even make it halfway through the salad, and my faint explanation of the car accident; she didn't miss a beat.

"Was this 'friend' a homosexual? Are you a homosexual?"

Part of me didn't hesitate; the other part froze. He was. I was. Neither of us was officially out yet.

"Yes."

I sat there staring at the salad waiting for what she would say. Maybe, because I was friends with Sarah, she would be enlightened, or uplifted with empathy or understanding, and the biblical teachings she regurgitated in her classes everyday would suddenly seem trivial. But, as I looked around her home in the deafening age of silence, I found it believable that this woman had never had a gay friend in her entire life.

"God probably took him away from you before you could start an inappropriate relationship with him."

Are you fucking kidding me? As suddenly as the tears I had dressed my salad with came, they went away. With as much control as I could find without jamming the salad fork into her throat, I put the fork down on the table where I found it. I pushed myself out of my chair and left her to the entrees.

At the end of my Business & Economics class the following Monday, Joanne chased me down the hallway and informed me that Mrs. Amy took it upon herself to announce to my class, in my absence, that I 'needed prayers' because I was 'going through something' and was 'struggling with homosexuality.'

Unknowingly, Mrs. Amy had placed herself in a checkmate. Being friends with Sarah, I knew things about them. I knew things like how Mrs. Amy was taking cases of beer to Sarah at college regularly; her nineteen-year-old daughter, a college freshman. My mind was a volcanic flow of vindictive anger and rage. The next thing I knew I was in Mrs. Amy's office, her glass house of bibles and upstanding facade, standing in front of the door blocking her way out.

"Who the fuck do you think you are?"

She stammered between justifications trying to assure me that she was acting in my best interest in my severed relationship with God. Prayers work.

"Oh, shut the fuck up! Wouldn't it be a shame if anyone ever found out about your beer trafficking to Sarah's college?"

The calm water of justifications she was standing on began to rock, and wave, and she sank off her Christ-like sandals. She took the deepest, most hypocritical breath she ever took and began to fold. She began to cry. With her head down, this tall, white-haired woman frantically began to apologize.

"You are not sorry for anything other than getting caught. Don't fuck with me."

My hand nearly slid off the doorknob as I whipped it open and swiftly escaped, leaving her in her shattered glass house. I couldn't decide if I wanted to laugh, cry, scream, or sprint home.

As I walked down the hall to my locker, my awareness of being stared at was heightened. Did they know? They knew. With my entire class being only thirty-three students in a four-hundred-person school, it seemed inconceivable that, in the ten minutes from last period to now, anyone was left uninformed.

When I got home, I threw my things on my bed and walked into the bathroom locking the door behind. I began to fish for the tweezers in the top drawer next to the sink. Not even out of my Catholic school uniform, the metal tongs, like a sewing machine, poked at my brow. Within minutes, my eyebrows, or what was left of them, were shaped, plucked, and preened within an inch of their life.

Shortly after the exchange with Mrs. Amy, Father Paul called Mother at work, keeping her on the phone for twenty minutes, informing her of what a terrible parent she was.

I regretted that, specifically the eyebrows, additionally the whole thing.

In the short period of time, it took me to respond to Mother, I enlisted in a nostalgic life-flashing-before-my-eyes journey to the past.

My parents basically went broke helping me move to and stay in The City. I regretted that.

In the second grade, I had the shit kicked out of me on the playground, which displaced Jeanie, Crissy, and I in our little Catholic school that Mother and Father paid for. I regretted that.

Mother and Father wouldn't let me take gymnastics at the local YMCA when I was six years old.

I had totaled my car in an accident that wasn't my fault and folded the hood of my new car in an accident that was. Three thousand dollars later, I regretted that.

At sixteen I was hired at Dorney Park in their disco review and quit my job as a glorified bus boy at the Hershey Hotel to do the show and live with a stranger in the Allentown area. They fired me four days before rehearsals; before I had even met the cast. I regretted that.

I stopped playing basketball after the ninth grade. I regretted that.

Even though grandma bought me tap shoes she found at a garage sale and offered to pay for tap lessons I never took dance. I regretted that.

I gave up the saxophone after six years.

I got bored with piano.

I never took guitar.

I regretted that. But nothing seemed to matter enough to count, and this wasn't confession, and Mother wasn't a priest, thank God.

"Not a one! No regrets at all."

I couldn't tell if Mother was shocked or relieved by my answer. She didn't say anything. She just smiled her small, quiet smile. Maybe she was expecting me to list off grievances that had subliminally ruined my life or damaged my psyche. But if there even were any, my child eyes didn't register them as worthy grievances. Perhaps she was thinking of instances that stuck out to her, but I wouldn't have noticed.

What I did notice was the ribcage and hipbones now visible through my thin, empty skin, in the mirror. I had never seen them before. Who knew I even had them?

THANKS CANCER!

25 Where There Never Was a Hat

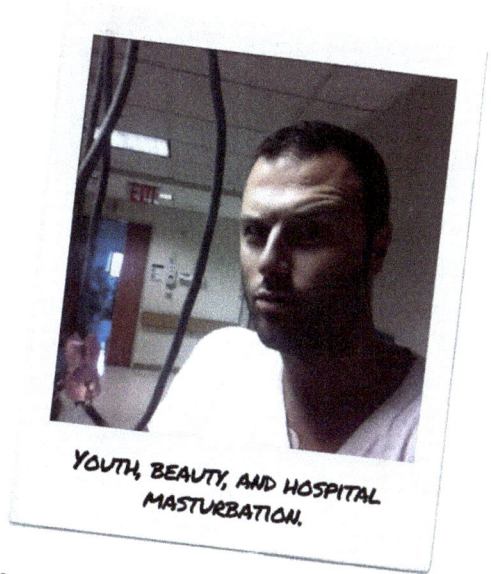

YOUTH, BEAUTY, AND HOSPITAL MASTURBATION.

The modest pile of large lumberjacks crawled over, and around me, their beards and chest hair dripping sweat, and spit all over my tensed-up body as they, and I took turns entering and exiting each other. I breathed in and out in rhythm with the nearly violent thrusts of the tattooed arms and hulking legs, as attention was paid to every inch of the inked mound of men. The force from which I was being taken by matched that of which I was giving. The brawn behind me wrapped his hefty arms around my chest and torso, placed his hand on my jaw, and turned my face around for mouth-to-mouth resuscitation. The smell of their fluffy dewy beards; the cleanliness of soap, the sexiness of citrus beard oil, the odor of exertion, made my entire body sing with A-Tonal grunting, and accelerated the percussive smacking of wet skin, and mouths, and other things.

"Mister Miskie? It's time to take your vitals."

Reluctantly, from the casual sleep-like position I jolted myself into as Nurse Phila opened the door, I positioned myself on my back, hiding the sad excuse for a pants-tent. This routine of random mid-night checks to make sure I hadn't spontaneously combusted was growing rather old, rather quickly.

"Oh my god, are you ok?"

The dampness on my forehead was a giveaway. She must have known what I was doing. The jig was up.

"Yeah. I'm fine. Aside from constantly being woken up."

167

Her shadow against my face hid the smile I was flashing her as the alarm in her voice rose. She grabbed my arm and placed her pointer, and middle finger on the inside of my wrist for three point four seconds.

"Your heartbeat is elevated and you're sweating. If you have a fever... We are going to have to do some blood work."

Oh, for fucks sake. I was jerking off and you interrupted my window of happiness. Let's not call in the big guns for the big gun. I was breaking some transplant rules and you caught me. Let's move on. She wouldn't move on. I was not going to tell her that she broke into my lumbersexual Bacchanalia, but she wasn't letting up. She jammed the plastic covered thermometer under my tongue, waiting for the telltale beep to trigger her next move.

"There's no fever, but I'm going to draw blood just to be safe."

Goddamnit!

By now, any sign of what little excitement I could muster had eradicated. Nurse Phila was teetering the line of calm and emergency, tightening the rubber tourniquet around my arm; I was somewhere between crying and laughing.

"Are you sure you don't feel fatigue? Ill? Nauseous?"

Seriously?

"Fatigue, yes, because no one here seems to want to let me sleep, otherwise, I feel amazing."

Collecting the tubes of blood, she had just let out of me, she assured me she would be back to let me know if they found anything irregular.

"Can't wait!"

The door closed behind her taking her false alarm along with her, leaving me to celebrate my being alone again. But should I?

Aside of the catastrophe I had infused into a nurse's night shift, Dr. Gloriosus's advice kept creeping into the fantasy of mountaineers I was mountaineering.

"DO NOT MASTURBATE!"

I asked this time around.

His voice motivated my movements, even through the warnings of bruising, brain hemorrhaging, internal bleeding, hernias, and hemorrhoids; the immediate outcomes of out-cum. Nurse Dot, from Manhattan County Hospital, her thick, stern accent, encouraging me to let it happen, soon accompanied his voice. In tandem of each other, their voices weaving in and out of the chest hair and beards I was summoning, devouring me in my head telling me no, telling me yes, telling me no, telling me God yes!

My toes began to curl, wrapped in the sheet, which had now inched its way down around my knees. My breath began to quicken, and grow deeper, and heavier. The muscles in my face began to contract and contort while the internal sneeze prepared itself to engage and expel itself. I muffled a heavy grunt behind my clasped and pursed lips. My face felt like it was going to erupt off my head. And just when the smatterings of dots were about to hit the canvas, the writhing of my insides produced a dull, quick, and staccato pain where the last of the lumberjacks had pulled out. Something swelled, or filled up, or exploded just outside of my inside gate.

Fuck.

Ouch!

Fuck!!!

Panting, I let go of the Polish Italian in case that was next to implode. Heaving in pain, I lay there concerned about my exit-entrance. It felt like someone had tried to shove a baseball bat into me with no lube, and no warning. Shit, this was bad. If this, whatever this was, was the start of another complication that was going to lead to a postponement of my discharge from this fucking transplant, I was going to lose it.

Again, the opposing instructions of Nurse Dot, and Dr. Gloriosus throbbed their way through the swell that now found itself just outside of me. I panicked. I half expected there to be blood everywhere by the time Nurse Phila returned to the room with my benign blood results. Surely this couldn't be serious. Surely, I didn't injure myself to the point of extending my hospital stay. Masturbation should not prompt a mental spiral into medical demise!

Finding the courage to reach down and inspect what this new dull discomfort could have been I hoisted my knees up just enough to let a little air in.

WOOF! FUCK! OUCH!

The throbbing swelled. I moved my hand down and employed a single digit to inspect the situation. Was I bleeding? Did I break it? Was something hanging out of it? Feeling around for the normal sort of texture, I ran into an abnormality that seemed somewhat like a small cherry, just to the right of center. Shit, shit, shit, shit. Self-diagnosing to the best of my ability, I deciphered, or at least assumed, that I had given myself a hemorrhoid. Masturbating... in a hospital... in the middle of a stem cell transplant. Perfect. Can't wait to explain this one to the nursing staff. Embarrassing!

I was so mad, so disappointed in my hemorrhoid and myself. How could this even be a thing? So, I deflected and came up with the best justification and excuse for having a random hemorrhoid I could think of. As Nurse Phila reentered the room, a few minutes later with my blood results that yielded no alarm, I told her I needed some hemorrhoid cream.

"Why do you need that?"

I was jerking off...

"I pooped too hard."

26 Into the Woods & Out of the Woods

It had been twenty-one days since my check-in at Sloan Kettering, and eleven consecutive days of isolation. My blood cells had finally lifted their heads to the heavens and begun to climb out of the chemo fissure they'd fallen into. My hemorrhoid was gone. There were no signs of the transplant failing. I was about to be set free. Set free into the next one hundred days, a period of required, utmost caution, as it was a bracket of time where the most could go wrong with my new, infantile immune system.

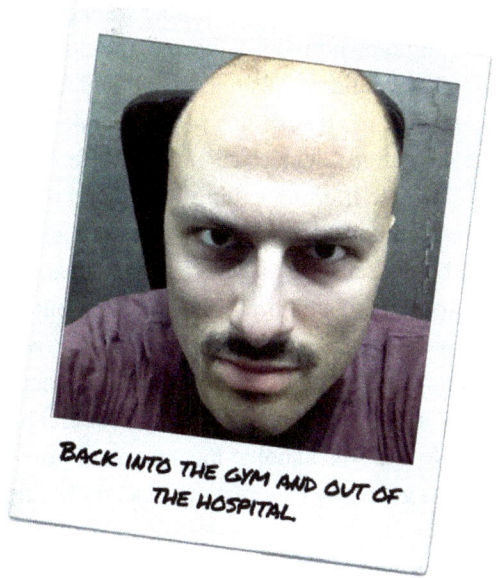

BACK INTO THE GYM AND OUT OF THE HOSPITAL.

No one had come into my room without a gown, facemask, or gloves in days. I hadn't seen a whole face for over a week. I hadn't walked more than ten feet in over a week. I hadn't taken a shower more than twice the whole time I was checked in; I wasn't allowed to. I was finally able to open the door to the hallway. I was in the clear and granted the go-ahead from Dr. Gloriosus to go.

As Mother and I waited for my discharge papers, the impatience I felt to leave was so strong I began to get angry. Hospital cabin fever is real. I stood in the open doorway of my corner room longingly looking over to the central nurse's station. As usual Mother was cool and calm in her chair.

"What's taking so long?"

Finally, Nurse Philia swaggered her way down the hall in my direction with a stack of papers in her manicured hands.

"Sign these, and these are for you, and you're all set."

I signed some papers. I checked out. I charged down the hall towards the elevators I had passed a few hundred times in our laps around the floor. They were the only things I wanted. Mother trailed behind, a little less feverish to leave, carrying one of my bags through the floor that had been my home for just shy of a month. The glamorous nurses that had tended to me, the patient with three kids and Leukemia, the chorus line of resident doctors, Dr. Gloriosus were all left behind in the dust of my clean escape back to life.

Back to life. Something I had spent the year anticipating as I watched my blood counts go up and down like the emotions that coursed through me, like the chemo, and blood transfusions, and antibiotics, and other prophylaxis. But as I dragged my backpack, bag, and tired, atrophied ass out of the hospital, I realized exactly how burnt out I was having barely moved for twenty-one days being flushed full of toxic waste. It occurred to me that I was not going back to life at all, at least not as I knew it before. There was no magical escape hatch to drop me off where I had left off. No one was handing me a guide or how-to book on what to do next. All I could do was get in the cab, rest my head on Mother's shoulder, catch my breath, and go home.

Stumble-jogging through the lobby of my new apartment building, panting after exhausting myself out of the taxi, Sakarian, the Eastern European doorman stood up, alarmed at the speed of my pace and alien-like figure that was infiltrating the hallway, and tried to stop me. No one was going to block me from my coveted apartment and bed. No one! Maybe he thought I was some sort of terrorist. It was July 2012, the hottest summer on record, and I was in a hoodie and a fur hat. If you see something say something?

"Hey. Hey! Where are you going?"

I didn't stop. Mother was behind me carrying my bag. My heartbeat was pounding in my chest like seventy-six trombones and a marching band.

"I live here!"

Barking at the doorman nearly toppled me over simultaneously tripping on the carpet runner: instant karma for being an asshole. Recovering from my falter I leaned up against the wall and smashed my hand onto the 'UP' elevator button. Mother and I ascended to the apartment I already missed. Father answered the door with blue rubber gloves and a mask on holding a ceramic knife in his right hand.

"Father, I'm ok, you don't have to wear those anymore."

He insisted. The studio apartment overwhelmingly smelled of gourmet food, or at least gourmet comparatively to that of hospital food. Though Sloan was leaps and bounds above Manhattan County Hospital in many departments, including food, it was still hospital food, lacking most seasoning and some of its flavor. They called it 'macrobiotic', which seemed to be cancer-talk for 'tolerably flavored.'

Father had spent the day cleaning the apartment Mother and he had hauled my belongings one hundred blocks downtown to move me into. The Fairway bags in the granny push-kart Father had bought at Bed, Bath, and Beyond, were filled with pre-approved groceries from a list Sloan had provided. The pop and sizzle of the salmon steak in the skillet was a welcomed ambiance from the sizzle of the central air at Sloan.

I collapsed face first on the actually comfortable bed by the window opening one eye for a moment to see if any of my new neighbors were up and at 'em in the afternoon sun. No one, just my parents ambling with purpose around the studio apartment, unpacking and setting up shop for the next very cautious one hundred days.

26.1 On the Steps of the Palace

I woke up to freedom, and the sun, and smells and breakfast. Everything hurt. It felt as if I'd annihilated my body at the gym the day before when in fact all I had done was carry my luggage out of the hospital and get out of a taxi. I hadn't even seen the inside of a gym for about two months, but the soreness and stiffness were comparable.

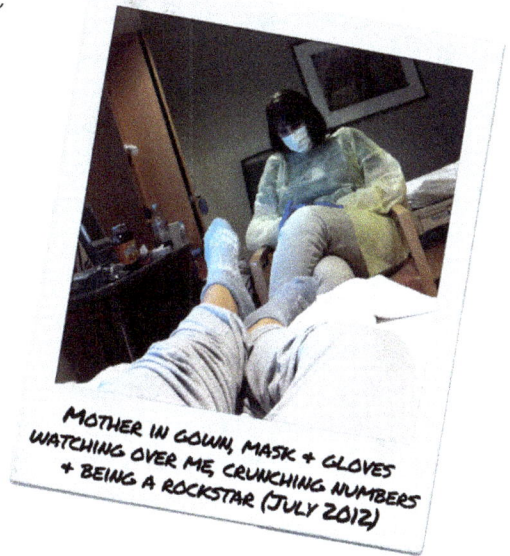

MOTHER IN GOWN, MASK + GLOVES WATCHING OVER ME, CRUNCHING NUMBERS + BEING A ROCKSTAR (JULY 2012)

Outside, it was gorgeous. The sun was shining without a cloud in the sky, and I had the option to go experience that. Inside the AC was kicking. Father stood over the hot plate in my counter-top kitchen scrambling eggs with the utmost of focus and care. I rolled over through the strain of the missing muscles all over my frail, pasty body greeting him and the day, the first day. Keeping the comforter wrapped around my unclothed form as I sat up cross-legged in bed, Father brought over my favorite breakfast: egg and cheese on a toasted English muffin.

"We're walking to the park today."

My parents had promised me they wouldn't let me sit around and be tired. I wanted to approach the next one hundred days with the same vigor I had approached cancer: like nothing was wrong. I had force-fed myself for months, and now it was time to force move myself, even if someone else was barking at me to do so, even if I was keeling over one foot in front of the other.

Hunched over my plate and the last bite of breakfast, I prepared myself to stand and walk the twenty feet to the shower. Placing my feet on the ground and my hands on either side of my legs, I pushed off the bed, still cloaked in blankets. Those twenty feet felt like a mile.

The hot water trickling down my back was like a giant hug that I sorely needed. The loud applause from the rising steam behind the curtain, fogging the walls and the mirror, was like a welcome home salutation from the shower nozzle. Vigorously, I shampooed my bald head with a minty wash. The tingling of the shampoo was so refreshing I barely noticed that I had rendered myself out of breath from the back-and-forth motion of my arms, lathering soap on my hairless scalp and body. Short of breath, I began to fade.

My surroundings became spotty and blurred as this sudden blackout set on. I braced myself on the towel rack at the back of the shower stall, my head between my arms, and my heels against the front of the tub. Inhale. Exhale. Only a few short moments passed before I came-to, still bent over the towel rack. So, this is where I was: winded from moving my arms. I grabbed a towel and slowly, as to not repeat the blackout, dried off.

Barely able to hang on to what was left of me, my bath towel clung for dear life onto the thighs and butt I once had. The mirror was an unkind word, from what should have been a friend, giving me the real run-down of the last few weeks. Somehow the hospital mirrors told a different story of how far I had gone, but at home, the mirror above the sink, placed not quite high enough to see my full face, was a harrowing tale. It seemed I had gone from Micheline, Kentucky Fried Chicken, porker to bouncing back radiation recovery story, to near cadaver in what seemed to be a single night. Nearing eight months since chemo one, it looked as though any traces of me had been flushed.

There couldn't have been more than a dozen hairs clinging desperately to the center of my chest. Like drapes, the swoop and droop of my skin had given me deflated breasts and wrinkly balloon arms and thighs. I wanted to cry, I wanted to scream and punch the mirror like I used to as a kid when the sobering realization that I was four times the size of my friends would set in, in the form of class photos and birthday party pictures. Instead, as I brushed my teeth and watched my limbs wobble and tremble in my toothbrush's momentum, I got angry - motivated.

"Ready?"

Hung over from the man in the mirror, I stood feet away from the glass door just inside the front of my building. Father was next to me ready for my first day in the Upper West Side as this recreation of science. The humidity of the outside clashed with the frigid, air-conditioned lobby each time someone else had the courage to open the front door and walk outside, but not me. Even though I had struggled through the simple task of getting dressed, my new purple shoes on my feet, I stood there next to Father looking at the sidewalk wandering if could handle the elements and my new-found inabilities. But the images of my crumpled up, trash-bag body kept re-reflecting on the glass doors in front of me, and I threw my determined weight into the handle and pushed open the glass.

Riverside Park was humming with dogs walking their persons, birds singing through the thick of summer, and the trees rustling in the faint breeze off the Hudson. Father and I followed the only, but unfamiliar path through the park entrance. Curving past the dog run, and into a tunnel, we were left dusted with kicked up gravel at the top of a humungous, nearly impossibly large staircase leading down to the riverfront.

This staircase looked as if it should have been connected to a palace. I half expected to reach the bottom and be met with a horse and carriage. Could I do this? I stopped to take stock. I had to decide, so I approached the stairs, casting a long shadow down the first flight, and began to take them to task. But only a few short stairs downwards, I was spent. White knuckling on the black railing, I cautioned my weight through my wrist. Father looked back to make sure I hadn't collapsed on the way down. Every few feet there were landings, and as each stone landing approached, I stopped, stuck. My feet were glued to the platforms, seemingly unable to continue. The shoes I was wearing felt heavy, as if my foot would have slipped right out of them.

Gathering myself back together, I continued as if I were on a deadline or escaping from something; cancer, myself, a prince? All four landings came and went. I stole a moment to heave through the heat, filling my lungs with summer, river air, and determination. Finally solid ground met my shoes, I made it. I didn't die, I wasn't stuck on the steps in my shoes. Father and I celebrated as we continued on to the green benches that lined the bike path along the Hudson.

Ankles crossed and my hands supporting me on the edge of the bench, Father and I sat there enjoying the non-hospital surroundings. He was always one for serenity and enjoyment of the peace and calm of nature, absorbing the sound of the Hudson River crashing against the cement island border. I was enjoying the gym shorts jogging by and the flop and shifts happening inside of them as their owner's legs hit the pavement.

The fire in my legs from the stairs had now moved to a more centralized location, reminding me that I could feel, but not function and my envy grew not only of the passerby's perky gear, but their ability to stride by like gazelles and wild horses. I wanted that. I wanted to be able to do something more than walk down a flight of stairs without traumatizing my body. The runners, and the bikers, and even the walkers proved to be another gigantic mirror of all the things I couldn't do or be.

"I'm ready to go."

This wasn't the joyous slipping-back-into-normalcy-welcome-home-reception-to-life I expected. It was like going to see Laura Benanti in a Broadway show, and after you've already paid for the ticket, took your seat, and the curtain rose you find that her understudy, who happened to be Fantasia Barrino, was on for her instead.

The unrealistic idea that I was going to be birthed out of the hospitals canal and bounce right back to where I was a year ago, married to the image of me in the mirror, and the glass door in the lobby, and runners, was infuriating. I felt deceived by myself, by the hospital, and by any cultural misunderstanding of what life after cancer was like. This was more taxing than any treatment or indecency I had undergone. Getting myself back was going to be an uphill, or rather up stair climb, but at least those steps of the palace were pretty to look at. As I clawed my way back up the stairs, heading home, Father behind me should I fall, climbing the steps of the palace, my purple shoe came off my foot, stuck to the hot stone steps.

26.2 Agony

Weeks of blanched tomatoes and egg sandwiches mundanely slumped by to where, if I had to eat one more fucking mushy vegetable or poached salmon, I was going to scream. Eating became agony, but short progresses were being made, and I had gruelingly graduated from winding myself in showers and stairs, to making my way down to the rickety fitness center in the basement of my building. In my first tank top of the summer, and the same pair

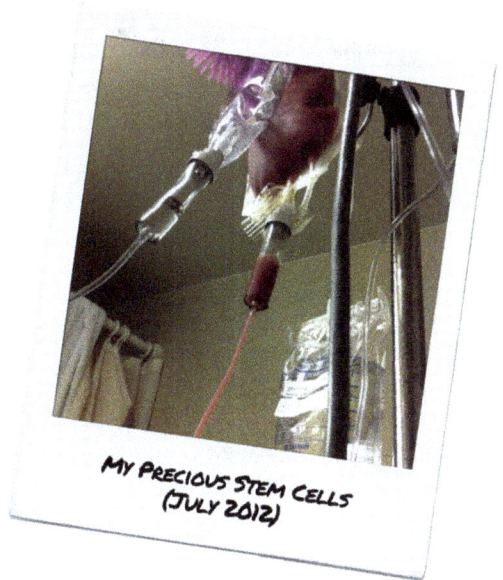

MY PRECIOUS STEM CELLS
(JULY 2012)

of basketball shorts I had been working out in for years, I stood in front of the wall-length mirrors trying to hold grip on twenty-pound free weights. I hadn't even curled them yet and my arms were already burning as if I had just pumped out a hundred preacher curls. The five minutes of low resistance, grandpa's pace, elliptical I knocked out moments prior, drenched me. My tank top sticking to my body cluing me in as to how shamefully aware I was of my missing stamina.

I glared at the man in the mirror angrily, who so pathetically could barely hold onto the little weights he was holding. Dustings of a familiar face misted across his glistening dome head and brow with a hint of fire behind his sullen, not yet defeated eyes.

This person in the mirror had betrayed me. He had betrayed me like my body had betrayed me and given me unexplainable cancer. He betrayed me like Beadle had, and Valentine had, leaving me on the starting line exactly when I needed him most. He was a wolf, a wolf in a freshly sheered sheep's clothing. All of this equipment in this sad little basement gym had betrayed me too.

Faint recollections of dominating these machines, reminding me that they used to be my friends and therapists, but now just sat there unattainable, taunting me like my elementary school peers used to taunt me for being a fat gay kid. Only now I was a full-grown adult barely revealing any improvement, and there was nothing I could do about it, but force and push myself.

Still locked into the eyes of this wolf in front of me, bending my knees just out of a lock, I inhaled the stale basement air, faint of its fitness attendees before me, and bore down on my core. Twenty pounds felt like a hundred and might as well have been with the way that my forearms and core were trembling under their weight. Holding my breath and pushing, morphing into that person at the gym that everyone hates, I howled out with each rep.

One!

"Hello, little girl!"

The wolf in the mirror taunted me yet didn't seem to be phased by my determination to rid myself of his presence.

Two!

"What's your rush? Take your time."

A mere five pumps upwards, I dropped them to the floor unable to maintain them any longer. Lightheaded and frustrated, having hoped that all of the walks to the river with Mother and Father weren't for nothing, I sat down on the bench-press, and slumped forward onto my knees. There, the wolf looked back at me in the mirrored walls, flashing his teeth. I called him off.

"There's no possible way to describe how I feel."

I had had it. It was time to leave the woods. Determined to prove that the wolf didn't stand a chance, I hired an instructor to come over once a week and force me into various positions for, what I lovingly called, 'naked yoga.' This prince of a man would speak under his breath in hushed relaxing tones that were sometimes lost under the grumble of the window unit. He was charming. He would guide me; touch me, like we were dancing. Unlike the leper that I felt like, this man didn't seem to be bothered by my physical state. And despite that I was paying him to impose my body into positions it was not acclimated to, nor ready for, his bare hands were welcomed on my naked skin. It felt wonderful, royal, new, almost. His lush voice and soft hands would guide my every move, and I could escape from my reality. Escape that I couldn't afford these sessions that I so looked forward to in the first place, or that I had no job, and no real income, and was unable to do anything about either of those things.

"Roll your hips up towards the sky and straighten your legs, pushing your heels towards the floor."

Eventually, I hit the bottom of the barrel and couldn't afford to pay the prince anymore. I let the moment go, but continued dancing in my apartment without him. I wasn't going to give up on me.

Edward Miskie

26.5 The Greens

As late September fell from the trees, I was left to stand on my own two feet without the watchful eyes and assistance of Mother and Father. Progress aside, I'd still wake up in a jolt needing a few minutes to realize I wasn't in the hospital; that the beeping of the garbage trucks outside weren't chemo pumps filling me with poison, that I was safe, and home. The pops and cracks that my body now produced, as I got out of bed, reminded

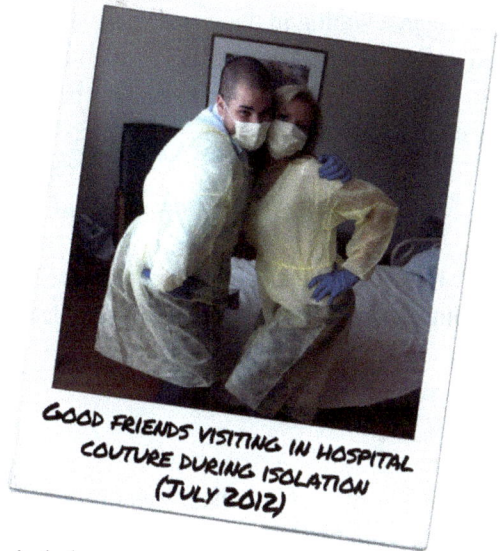

GOOD FRIENDS VISITING IN HOSPITAL COUTURE DURING ISOLATION (JULY 2012)

me of the pop and clicks of the port tubes, heaving me down a temporary hole I'd have to breathe, and concentrate to get myself out of. I'd hold onto my sheets, and my coffees, and showers as clear indicators in my mornings that I was not still locked up in a hospital room.

Still the days progressed, though beautiful and sunny, they still demanded proof that I was free. Not leaving my apartment became a trigger for anxiety, and I'd have to calm myself down by walking outside and leaving for hours. If I wasn't out and about by 11am some days, I was a mess.

Early evening rolled around, and I had made my way back to the apartment after a long walk around the neighborhood. I was finally independent enough to familiarize myself with the outside, deterring from the path to the Hudson in Riverside Park. Sakarian greeted me at the front door, and I walked around the corner to the mailboxes to check the post. The initial $3,500 Mother had paid outright to Manhattan County Hospital at the demands of Thenardier, finally showed up: a reimbursement check.

I couldn't believe it. After nearly a year, and literally, after one hundred phone calls, after chasing down account managers, after constantly hounding the insurance company, and the hospital, and the credit card company, after more paperwork was demanded, submitted, lost, and resubmitted, the check arrived. But the check arrived with my name on it because I was the patient. Even though I was not the credit card holder, the check was made out to me. I looked at it, and that number, and I pined, fantasizing of all I could do with that green. What I wanted more than anything in the world was the green! It was the missing piece. My hair had grown back, curly, and dark. I'd gotten my footing back and could walk, even jog. Food I was not allowed to eat was becoming scarce. I was starting to fill out my clothes, again.

"Just deposit it into your account and when it clears, send me an online check."

Mother's suggestion, depositing the check that definitely, rightfully belonged to her, into my account was like asking an alcoholic to go to a bar and hold your drink.

"Alright!"

But it wasn't, quite. There was freedom in that check. All my problems would be solved with that one piece of paper. There were three months of disability pay in that check. If it wasn't bad enough that I had lost my sense of worth, I had also lost my actual worth. Savings had run out shortly after Christmas and trickled into phone calls to parents and grandparents for help before paperwork for any benefits could be processed. Even that took months too long.

Curled up on my bed, having deposited the check on my bank app, holding the useless stub, I fell asleep, only waking up to find that I had full-out moved to snuggling the check. I was big spooning the green, or a memory of having it. Once the check cleared into my account I lovingly and longingly looked at the numbers. I could barely remember the days of having savings stocked up from working on ships, or what I could scrounge together living on the road. Would I ever get back to that? To the life of gallivanting from town-to-town, putting a show up in two weeks, and living off nothing to pack away as much as I could to come back to The City with? To audition! Did I miss that? Was I sure? Did I want that again? I supposed it was too soon to tell.

Begrudgingly, with a twitch of bitterness, knowing it was the right thing to do, I sent off an online payment to Mother totaling the full amount. This spell was on my house! Somehow, I would figure it out.

27 I'm Still Here

October 5th, 2012. My 26th Birthday was two days away and I had made a reservation for ten at KTCHN on West 42nd Street. The tone of this birthday, a birthday none of the ten were completely sure I was even going to have, was going to be widely affected by the results of the day. It was a Friday and I had been up, unfed, and uncoffeed since seven in the morning. The one hundred days were up, and I was headed for Sloan Kettering for the appointment that really counted. I had one more thing to do: get through the day.

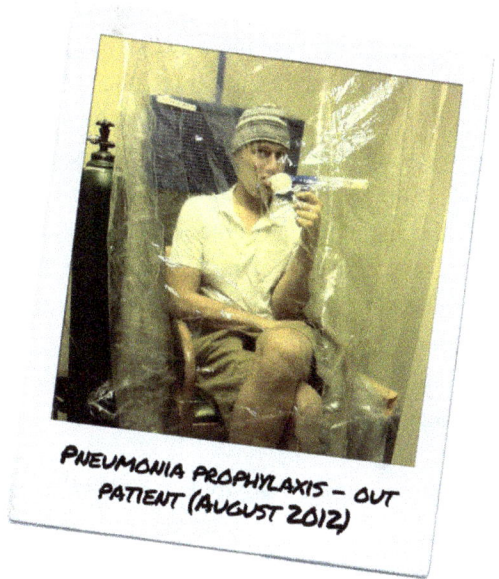

PNEUMONIA PROPHYLAXIS - OUT PATIENT (AUGUST 2012)

"Sorry to keep you waiting. I'm running a little bit behind. I'll be right in."

Goddamn it. My nerves were already thinning little ice crystals, and the abrupt closing of the door behind Dr. Anthony furthered the cracking process.

At this point in the calendar, most of this was all old hats; like a reunion that happened every few days. I'd start with blood work, move to a CT scan, and end up in an exam room waiting for Dr. Anthony to come tell me we were good... for now. For the last time as I knew it, I made my way into the exam room on East 64th Street waiting for the results. *The results.* The results that were going to determine if I was going to be shoved back into treatment, living on a hope and a prayer, or if I could make a plan, for a change, as to what I could do for the rest of the year. Hell, the rest of the week!

Anthony sat in a chair to my right, his elbows on his knees; his hands clasped together staring at the floor. I was so glad he was there. Foolishly I told my parents not to come in for a quick scan and appointment, but I really could have used them in the room. I brushed this appointment off as if it weren't a big deal to me. I was fine. It had been weeks since they had last come into The City to help me with the day to day, and I didn't need them anymore. Except I did, and I was now kicking myself for having kept them away.

It had been hours since my blood work was taken, and my CT scan was complete. My imagination had already gotten the best of me, and I was hallucinating ghosts of my patient-self walking around the room, wringing their hands at me waiting to drag my existence back into the hospital; into the past. I leaned up against the counter on the far end of the room gripping it as hard as I could, having to remind myself to inhale. I watched the staff photography fade in and out on the computers screen saver, until Dr. Anthony had popped her head into the door, giving us her tardy status.

Anthony and I froze in our already still positions as the exam room door swung open again, and Dr. Anthony peeked her head of curly hair back into the silence.

"Oh, and everything looks great! I'll be right back."

Don't Look at Me. I thought I was *Losing My Mind*. I had spent *Too Many Mornings* wondering *When Could I Leave You*, to send Seymour down the *Road You Didn't Take*. But now, I was assured that *You're Going to Love Tomorrow*, and suddenly I could *Live, Laugh, Love*.

The words came out of Dr. Anthony's mouth so matter-of-factly, and so flippantly, that it took me a second to register what she had said. Nothing had spread, and nothing new popped up. It was over! It was fucking over! The notion that I could now put this whole period of my life behind me was exhilarating; the biggest relief I've ever felt. Seymour had officially left my body, calming the chaos. Anthony and I looked at each other, and suddenly I could let go of the damn countertop and breath. He stood up and we hugged. I pawed at him as though I hadn't seen him in a decade, clinging onto him for life, quite literally for life. I was definitely crying. I was really free this time.

"Well. I'll see you in January for your next follow up! Congratulations!"

A quick exam, and well wishes from Dr. Anthony, and I was out the door, Anthony by my side, nearly skipping. We walked out of the automatic, double doors to the sidewalk. The sun was just about to set to a pink and orange sky, broken up only by tall buildings, and infrastructure. The City seemed beautiful again, like I had taken off the grey scale glasses, and saw everything as it really was; as I hadn't for a very long time.

Anthony bid me congratulations and farewell as the M72 bus pulled away from Third Avenue and 72nd Street to make its way West. All the silence and stillness of the last year, the uncertainty and palpable dread shed with each passing avenue. Like a second skin I'd been forced to wear for the past eight months, it peeled off, layer by layer in the breeze of Central Park, as the bus blew through to Broadway.

I leapt off the bus with a spring in my step, to the beat of the invisible orchestra pumping throughout the Upper West Side. All I wanted, was to sit in my apartment, in the quiet of my Upper West Side studio, and savor a pint of Ben & Jerry's. No more macrobiotic noodles, no more blanching tomatoes and peppers, no more, no more, no more! I wanted to order a pizza. I wanted to order sushi. I wanted to order every single thing I wasn't able to have for the last few months. But I settled for a pint of New York Super Fudge Chunk because fuck, yeah!

I kicked my feet up onto the corner of my desk with the pint in one hand, a spoon in the other, and my phone sitting on my desk on speaker. I called Mother and Father, Crissy and Jeanie, Aunt Phyllis, my grandparents and the pillar-friends who had sat with me through all of this.

"Seymour's gone. We're all good!"

After the phone calls were made, and everyone I needed to contact was called, I still had one more thing to do. I logged onto social media; the one place I had never dared utter the C word and began to pen the process of another coming out.

"For those of you who had any doubt in your mind as to how tough and how bad-ass I really am, I would just like to inform you all that I have officially beat Cancer (NHL). I will not be giving any details on this. Some knew, some didn't. I had it, it's gone; It's over and I'm still fuckin' here and I'll drink to that! Onwards and Upwards... I'm Still Here."

I gathered up a big pile of laundry and went to the basement. As I watched the last few minutes of the drier cycle push my clean clothes around in a circle, I smiled, knowing it was going to be a good birthday; I was going to have another birthday.

28 Ladies and Their Sensitivities

All of the familiar faces were out and about. Hugs and hellos were all the same, the lines were still horrendously long, the studios were still shoulder to shoulder crowded, and the faces of those in line still steadfast and unbending, the hold outs. It was February 2013, which only meant it was audition season once again; my first audition season back in the game since I had

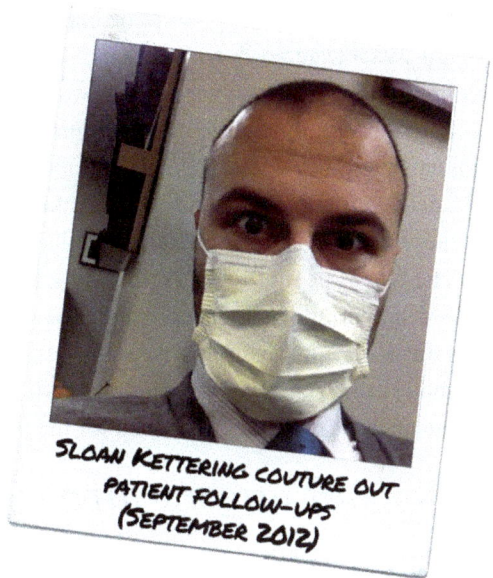

SLOAN KETTERING COUTURE OUT PATIENT FOLLOW-UPS (SEPTEMBER 2012)

been freed from the tight grasp of Sloan Kettering. Life was beginning to develop a rhythm that didn't make me miserable. Wake up, audition my ass off, gym, nap, work. Sometimes I'd throw in a midday happy hour just to take the heavy edge off the collective one hundred and twenty-eight bar audition days.

"Fuck this! I'm done! Let's get a beer."

But for the most part, I was excited to be back in a way that I hadn't been excited for a very long time. February is always an insane month for we musical theatre folk. Audition season officially bestows itself upon us and makes a routine out of early wake up calls and over caffeinating ourselves just to get to noon. If you're lucky you're finished around 1pm and can slink your way over to a dump of a bar for a cheap drink to numb the indecencies of the day, or celebrate the successes, all before work. But eventually, all of the days and auditions run together, and you can't remember whom you just auditioned for let alone what.

"I sang Carousel again."

"That audition was for Next to Normal."

"Great!"

Hard as it was, it felt good to be back, and with Ronnie by my side almost daily, it was a watered-down version of enjoyable. We sat inside the door of a holding room at Ripley Grier Studios waiting for our audition group to be called. Waiting for our moment of sixteen to thirty-two bars of 'hire me' to be up. I had been up since 5am, was on my fifth coffee, and was ready for a nap. It was now 1pm, and auditioning, as I had always joked was a 'full time job,' was looking more and more like a dead serious statement than a flippant remark.

The two of us sat in the black folding chairs and paged through our audition books deciphering what we were going to sing for this one: always the struggle. Does this song align with their season? Am I right for this show? If I sing this song, will they know what role or show I'm auditioning for? Do you think they'll remember the last time I auditioned for them and sang the same thing?

"GOD WHAT AM I GOING TO DO?"

I had a new book of songs to audition with to go along with the new me I was auditioning with, and even though the stakes were low being it was my first season back from cancer, I was still anxious. Ronnie and I swam amongst our high-end plights, air-drying from the rain outside. We vacillated from page to page of our books, chirping along with the rest of the dampened excitement of the room, when a presence caught my attention and tugged my ear towards the front door. It was a familiar voice, a tambour I recognized and engaged my brains sense memory.

Shit.

I could tell something was, not wrong, but off. It was a hair of a second but peering over to the monitor's table I knew it was him. Double taking, seeing the back of a big, tall, curly dark-haired man, I had no doubt in my mind - it had to be. I whipped my head back over to Ronnie and dug my knuckle into his knee giving him a big wide eyed 'oh shit' face. My lower lip pulled down to the right side of my jaw having only one reaction to the unavoidable awkwardness that just walked in the room: Beadle.

The two of us had not shared the same oxygen since radiation; since I'd run into him outside of my gym and he informed me, after talking his way through my problems back to him, that he moved in with his partner and everything was going so grand and wonderfully in his life. Though somewhere deep down I felt safe. He was a WASP, family money, unable to actually have external unpleasant thoughts or feelings whatsoever. I was counting on him buttoning up the second he realized I was there and keeping his glances to his audition book, or the wall, or the floor; anything. The last time I attempted to reach out to him was rather embarrassing on my end, so I was kind of planning on doing the same. It had been about a year, but the drunken voicemail I left him while he was on vacation with his partner and family wasn't something I'd soon like to remember or discuss.

Definitely regretted it shortly thereafter, and again now, I played the voicemail back to myself in my head and felt so silly, so stupid, but so confident that he wouldn't want to cause a scene or speak to me. I couldn't help but wonder what would happen should I just walk up to him and inform him that I was still alive, much to his negligence and, or surprise. I brushed it off and forgot about it, much as I could with him sitting ten feet away.

"Yikes."

Ronnie returned the 'yikes' face, unabashedly watching Beadle stomp past us dripping rain from his coat with every important step. A droplet hit my hand, my knee. Unsure if he had seen us when he turned around from the front table, unsure if it mattered, but how could he not have seen us? We were right there. I'm a huge human, and Ronnie is loud. Surely, he would have noticed us at the very least, even if by accident. Forget it. Never mind, it's fine, it's fine, it's fine. I put the thought out of my mind and returned to flipping through my audition book with Ronnie, keeping Beadle in my conscious periphery just in case.

Minutes passed and I had forgotten about the whole thing. The room began to get muggy. This was not helped sitting amid the gaggle of chatty actors, afraid to leave the room should we miss our names being called and face being ejected from the audition list. We stayed, and steamed under the harsh fluorescents, and filled the room with hot air. Even with a window open, a window whose frame was now glazed with a layer of condensation, the air was thick and tepid to breath in. I sat there trying to focus on Ronnie and our antics, my audition book, my outfit; back in the saddle, was it all lining up? I was uncomfortable all around, feeling out of place, to an extent, despite all the familiar audition regulars. I grew more and more sensitive in the muggy room to any concentrated heat on my body, my knee.

I half expected to turn my head and see a friend connected to the hand that now rested on my right knee. Ronnie and my conversation derailed. Ronnie giving no sign or signal to the fact that Beadle had slinked his way over to where we were seated, bent his six-foot-four frame down, and placed his hand on my knee with a familiar smug look on his pinched face. It wasn't intentional; it was just how he looked. I looked at Ronnie, Ronnie looked at Beadle, I looked at Beadle, who was bouncing between looking at the both of us.

"You know, you're going to have to talk to me eventually."

Ronnie sat there silent, holding his breath, unsure of what I was about to do. All I could do was laugh. If I hadn't laughed, I probably would have either screamed or just walked out of the room. By now I had already mourned the loss of this friendship and despite some residual anger, was maybe at peace with it? But this sense of certainty, which surrounded my hesitance for everything else, reared its head at me. Even though I felt like I was clueless in the audition department, was terrified on a daily basis of any little cough, bruise, or abnormality, turning back into Seymour, one thing I did know, and I was completely confidant that the last year had taught me, was who my friends were. By all outward signs and definitions considered, this was not one of them.

I focused on his hand on my knee. He was touching me. He was touching me like a person of familiarity would do if they came up to you at a party and said hello or hugged you. For a second it brought back audition days of yore, signing each other up, hanging out in the holding room, going for coffee or lunch afterwards with Anthony. For a second it made me miss him, though he stood right there. It made me remember how much fun we used to have at my going away parties any time I'd leave town, or get-togethers I'd host whenever I came back. There was this one time at Landmarc, what a fucking good time, but now I was curious if he only came along because I offered to pay with the ship money I had just disembarked to land with. I didn't know who this person was anymore, or I wasn't sure. In fact, he had become quite the stranger; disinterested in what was going on in my life, and in reciprocity, I in his.

Fighting between heartache, fear, and anger, I had to face the reality that his opening line was 'you're going to have to talk to me.' That was the first thing he chose to say to me after months in which he ignored me, never having reached out once, knowing full well that I was living through the most terrifying experiences of my life. He was trying to put all of that on me. That I was going to HAVE to talk to him as if he were Ronnie, who bounced between my hospital and his mother's hospital while she was being treated for breast cancer. Or Anthony, or Senex who would come visit me several times a week just so I could have a body in the room, to not be alone. Or Grizabella, Dionne, Julie, Sheila, Berger, or the rest of the Tribe. Even Pirelli, who came home from Japan to see family and visit me. Beadle couldn't even return a text.

There were so many things I wanted to say. So many opportunities in this twelve-second span of me just staring at him with every consideration I had fluttering through my mind. I could have just let it all out and said all the things that I had wanted to for the last eight months; save that one voice mail. I could stitch the friendship back together, or let it go entirely, burning the bridge between his hand and my knee. But instead, I just sat there clutching my book of music, damp from the thickness of the room's atmosphere and looked up at him.

"No. No, I'm really not."

Ronnie broke. He cackled right in Beadle's face and mine. It was so out of place in the low tremor of hopefuls in the room. I almost apologized. I didn't know what to do. Never breaking eye contact, never making an intentional decision of how to react, Ronnie's trumpet-like chortle began to infect the muscles in my cheeks, and I began to smile; to laugh. I fought it, trying to tell myself 'No, no, no, no, don't do it!' But the nervousness and inappropriateness of the whole situation was too much, and I started to laugh.

Beadle's face, though I didn't think it was possible, grew more and more smug as he stood straight up from his prostrated position over me, removing his hand from my leg. Really, I felt bad and wanted to stop and say something else, maybe asking him for an apology, maybe suggest we go somewhere else and talk, but before I could level fighting off laughing long enough to say anything, Beadle took the wheel and that opportunity away from me.

"Fine! Fuck you very much!"

He stormed out of the room like a toddler who had his toys taken away from him, which made Ronnie laugh even harder. Had he even auditioned yet? I tried to keep smiling, brushing it off. I didn't care. No. What a jerk. How dare he, after all the time I had wasted on him being a friend. He lied to me from the start about even remotely giving a shit. Gross. What a jerk. My self-convincing planted a seed of doubt inside of me and drove it into the ground with each step Beadle took in the opposite direction.

Fuck me very much. That's all I got. That's it. It took me a minute to turn away from the empty doorway that Beadle had just walked out of. Numb to the fact that I was no longer smiling at all, not even a little bit. Ronnie, seemingly completely ignorant of my shift in mood, sighed out of his hysterics and readjusted himself in the folding chair.

"What the hell was that?"

I couldn't even answer that question if I tried. Ronnie's snickering faded with each shake of his head, and he dove right back into his music. Whether or not I felt empowered or defeated by the scene that was made, and the clean, or not so clean break of friendship was yet to be determined. Should I have gone after Beadle? I began to fantasize about what scene would have played out had I ran out after him and stopped him in the corridor just under the stairs. Perhaps I could have calmed us both down and talked it out; bought him a coffee? Assuming he would be receptive to anything I had to say in the first place, assuming he could put aside his lack of social graces and feigned politeness to have a no-nonsense discussion of where we stood. Had I made the wrong decision? Did I choose the wrong words? Was I too much of a bitch? Bitch on bitch fighting never ends in a peaceful negotiation, just tantrums or stomping away. I imagined him in the elevator, huffing and puffing his frustrations, or whatever feeling he was cultivating, away. Cursing my name? Wishing cancer had won?

But for the time being, in a room full of familiar strangers, I came to the realization that for the first time I didn't feel obligated to need a person. Something flicked on, or off, in my brain that reevaluated what I was getting out of that non-union. What I was getting out of what I called friendship verses what I was putting into it didn't make sense and suddenly 'fuck you very much' was just a door closing, cuing a window somewhere to open. Regretting not going after him, regretting what either of us had said in our exchange was useless at this point. He was probably walking through the rain up Eighth Avenue by now, pushing all of this down, en-route to his next audition. In fact, it occurred to me that by the time the elevator descended the sixteen floors and let him out into the gray lobby of 520 Eighth Avenue, he was probably already over it and moved on.

"Edward Miskie."

The audition monitor called my name to get in line. I still hadn't picked a song. Standing and taking off my sticky sweater, I quickly ripped off my wet Henley, threw on a button-down shirt and walked into the hallway, tacking myself onto the back of the line. Half-heartedly paying attention to the monitors instructions, still flipping through my book deciding what cut of sixteen bars I was going to sing, I stopped dead at the last song in the back of my book of music; the section of songs I don't use that often. It was perfect, it was so apropos, it made me laugh: "Ladies and Their Sensitivities".

29 My Body Is My Business

I came over for steak and eggs before I gave him my steak and eggs. Slick took my cleaned plate over to the kitchen sink as I waited in the dining room chair by the window. His apartment was one of the largest studios I'd ever seen; large enough to fit a king size bed and a round dining room table that sat four comfortably. As he rinsed off the breakfast plates, talking of supersets, weight increases, and diet regiments, I fell board, and my eyes

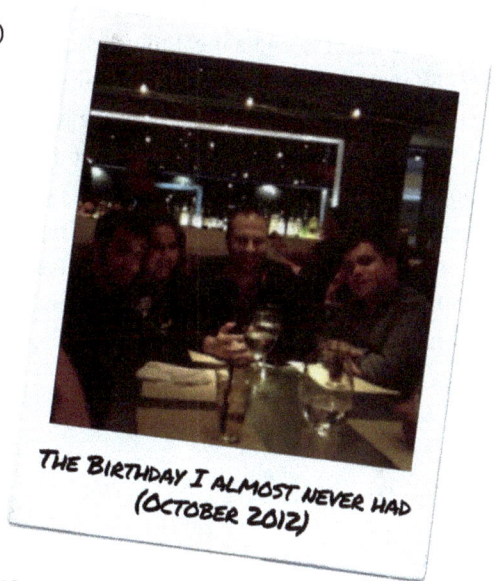

THE BIRTHDAY I ALMOST NEVER HAD (OCTOBER 2012)

fell on the plump scoops of ice cream that sat just below his back. How could this tall, chiseled, marble statue be into me at all? To be fair, he wasn't my typical type either, but whatever. He had taken me under his veiny wing at the gym I had joined and began to train me in exchange for a plowing. He'd make me squat and lunge and then I would make him squat and lunge.

In his standard gym shorts and tank top, Slick walked back across the wooden floors towards me, already pre-raised as indicated by the swing in his shorts. I, on the other hand, sat by the window wondering why there was no swing in my shorts. Encounters had been few and far between outside of my own indulgence to gauge the southern frontier. Slick reached down and picked me up under my armpits where Seymour used to be - ugh don't touch that - as he slid down to the floor, to his knees.

Grabbing me by the waistband of my gym shorts, he popped the Polish Italian out to freedom and claimed it as breakfast's dessert. As if I were lamenting an acting class exercise via A Chorus Line, I felt nothing. Well maybe not nothing, but damn near close to it as his face bounced off my unkempt nether regions.

Deflecting, and hoping he hadn't noticed, but fucking shit how could he not, I reached down and picked him up by the armpits and pseudo-aggressively shoved him towards the expansive king size bed. I was in charge here. Please disregard my hopefully temporary dysfunction. Making sure he couldn't see me, I positioned him on his knees on the edge of the bed, bent over, supporting himself on his elbows. I began to eat cake, though already full-on steak and eggs, but as a former fat kid, I never saw need to end a meal too early. I ate and tugged, and ate and rubbed, and ate and just short of shook it off. It still made it only to a half-mast position, which in my mind was just enough to get the job done.

Grateful that Slick, through his grunts and whimpers, couldn't see the nerves dripping down my face, the frustration pooling on the sheet underneath him, I began to slip and slide in, barely breaking through. But still, I made it in and feverishly began to thrust forward. My hands positioned on his meaty haunches, slamming them against my hips in search of any sensation or hope in graduating past half-mast, he had a different idea.

"Let me turn over."

FUCK!

NO!

The last thing I wanted were his abs and piercing blue eyes staring at me; judging me and my barely toned squash arms that hung from out my shoulder sockets, my valance gut that had picked itself up from drapes, but still wasn't immovable.

As he tossed himself on to his back, I flopped out and swung almost fluffed, but still not full. I grabbed it, hiding it from his line of vision, making sure he couldn't see the sad sauntering story between my legs. I could feel the heat of humiliation covering my sweat drenched, naked body as he fan-kicked his left leg over my head resting his heel on my right shoulder. All the while, I held the disappointing balloon in my left hand, casually hiding its discrepancy by ferociously yanking at it trying desperately to slap the shit out of it screaming to myself 'what the fuck is wrong with you?'

Hide. I should hide. My internal thought process redirected from trying to be successful at this farcical nonsense to mapping out the apartment for a place I could crawl into that was not a beef cake and die. I didn't need to work out that badly. I didn't need help at the gym after all. I was perfectly fine; in fact, I thought I could see an ab forming as I crammed the gelatinous form back into the pastry.

"OOFF! Careful."

Oh, God now I was hurting him. I was not only flopping around like a fish out of water, but now I was injuring him. I apologized through a charming smile hoping it masked the fact that I wanted to jump out of the floor to ceiling front window. I braced myself, using his ankles as leverage for the continued part two expedition for sensation and relief.

How could this be happening? Sure, cancer decimated my breakfast sausage, but I had done everything I could to keep it moving, as little movement as I'd get out of it. Why was I twenty-six years old and facing erectile dysfunction? Shouldn't the recovery process be far enough along for me to function like a normal human? It had been over six months since my birthday, and I was on the upswing, I was still young, and virile, and full of nuked sperm. Justifying this impossibility, jack hammering this marble statue as he played along with 'ooo's' and 'ahh's' on the white sheets, the whole charade felt gross, and I decided to abort and abort.

Having reached a point where I felt like neither of us could possibly, actually be enjoying ourselves, I pulled back. Resting on my heels and taking matters into my own hands, I frustratingly pulling on this goddamn useless mound of flesh. At long last, after soaking the sheets in shame, I soaked the sheets and Slick, in nuked babies. We both got up like nothing happened, mainly because not much did, toweled off in silence, and left.

After an ironically rigorous 'leg day' at Equinox on West 76th Street, Slick proposed we go for a coffee. The suggestion of which immediately made me assume that he was going to either bring up the lack of wind in my sails, tell me that this wasn't working out anymore, or both. Instead, we walked through the drizzly spring afternoon to Levain bakery. This is where the most addicting, delicious, and calorically driven cookies are sold.

"They're like, the size of a fist."

Why did we work out in the first place?

Walking down the stairs in the dense smell of Heaven, Slick and I approached to countertop covered in cookies and other such pastries.

"What can I get you?"

On the other side of the glass menagerie of chocolate trinkets was a bearded blond, much less difficult to look at, and much more on my level. Carting trophies around is exhausting. Slick took the wheel and ordered a chocolate chip, walnut, heaven devil cloud of a cookie for us to split, and two coffees.

Still in the current of my humiliatingly ill performance, the moment Slick left me to my half of the cookie and my coffee, not having said a word, I fired up my 'social app' in tandem to my apartment door closing. How had I not seen this handsome beardy before? His photo was right there on the grid of the neighborhood and its options. I immediately messaged him and started rowing the oars towards our first encounter. His name was Memphis.

I woke up in my apartment next to Memphis two weeks after our first meet-up, turned date, turned spending the whole day together. Over my shoulder I did a quick inspection of this fast and new installation into my life. I smiled at the idea casually swallowing, as one does, only to be yanked into nightmare territory. It hurt. There was soreness in my neck and throat that in the few seconds of morning I had been exposed to, could not explain. Placing my hands on my throat, to my terror I discovered one gland on either side of my trachea was swollen. I froze as I poked and rubbed them to make them go away.

During treatment I had contact with a woman whose husband died from a very similar type of cancer as mine. She once told me about the final days of her husband, and how in the end the cancer had gotten so bad and so aggressive that you could actually watch the tumors grow, specifically the tumors in his neck. It was happening. I was convinced. These glands had flared up overnight and despite my propensity for allergies, I had this sick sinking feeling that these were windpipe-crushing tumors. Panic equivalent to missing an alarm and being late for work tossed me out of bed leaping over Memphis, bounding towards the bathroom.

There they were, clearly visible in the bathroom mirror without any neck position manipulation. I could easily make out the almond shapes in my neck and I stopped breathing staring at them in the glass. This couldn't be happening. I was about to leave for Massachusetts to do The Sound of Music at North Shore Music Theatre. Not only was this theatre famed amongst actors for being incredible to work for, but this job was my first since the hospital. I was not going to miss this because Seymour decided to show up again, if he had decided to show up again. So, I spent minute upon minute inspecting these two lumps, swollen, and just shy of hard in pure panic-attack mode struggling to keep quiet as to not wake Memphis. They had to go away!

I had made it to Massachusetts, throat lumps in tow, and was completely mental in the thick of rehearsals. The hills were alive, and my glands had not shrunk. I sat buried in Rogers & Hammerstein compulsively pushing on and pressing my mini Seymours. With each passing Nun and Nazi, the fear swelled on and off stage. When I'd sing, they'd sing, when I spoke, they'd speak, and it became an exhausting routine to push down the hysteria.

I'd cry myself to sleep after rehearsals and performances, muffling the sounds in my pillow in cast housing so none of my neighboring cast mates could hear me. Fear had taken residence in my new life. I hated that I had gotten to that point because of a swollen gland, so instead of dealing with it, I discovered a guaranteed way to get myself to sleep through the living nightmare. Wine.

My show routine, even in the short four-week contract, quickly became a rotation of drinking myself to sleep at night and propping myself up during the day with pots full of coffee. I'd call Mother on breaks in a complete state of irrationality to say out loud over and over again that it was nothing, repeating constantly my final prognosis.

"Radiation killed Seymour, the Stem Cell Transplant finalized and nearly guaranteed a cure. Radiation killed Seymour, the Stem Cell Transplant finalized and nearly guaranteed a cure."

Nearly. 'Nearly' was what had me going. This dark cloud coated my every move, thinking about and inspecting what could come of this. Maybe if I don't touch it, it'll go away. Maybe if I stop talking about it, or thinking about it, they'll shrink? And by the time I had climbed every mountain for the last time, they did go away, and I went back to the city a little more fragile than I had left it.

Fresh out of Nazi Austria, I resumed life in The City for a time before I was set to leave for Florida to do Moon Over Buffalo. With not enough time between contracts to get a job, but too much time to do nothing, I went looking for some fun. Memphis and I were new, but not exclusive, and with the travel I had coming up I wasn't even sure if he would want to stick around. Dating as a traveling actor is tough like that. A couple, JoJo and Fleetwood, found me on the same 'social app' and began courting me with the idea of naked camp; a literal camp in the Poconos where one can frolic around the forest naked accompanied by a pool, a restaurant, and camp-like itinerary. Intrigued, but no. The idea of walking around naked in front of a bunch of strangers? I wasn't there yet.

Though the hair on my body had joined the hair on my head and face, having burst its way back across my chest and torso, and basically everywhere else, there was still a barren area on my left shoulder and pectoral where nothing grew. It looked ridiculous, like I was wearing a chest hair sash in a Miss Hairiest Beast competition. I hated it. Everyone commented on it taking me back to my middle school nickname: Boobs. Additionally, at radiations doing, the muscle growth on the left side of my chest was disproportionate with the right. Regardless of the left-heavy workouts and the favoring of that side when lifting, it was still fluffy and drooped noticeably lower than my right. Boobs.

Physically I still felt like a mutant and didn't want the pressure of walking around, balls out, in front of a pool full of judgmental naked homosexuals. But Fleetwood and JoJo insisted that it was not like that, and the experience as a whole was one not to be missed. They were leaving the next day, and I had to decide. So, we met for a beer at Candle Bar, just a block from my apartment, to make sure the other party wasn't an insane murderer.

In their rented SUV the following morning, Fleetwood and JoJo picked me up with their friend Snickers. Through New Jersey, into Pennsylvania, only stopping for booze and food, i.e., supplies for the weekend, JoJo turned over his left shoulder and smiled at me triggering a memory. Yes, we had gotten along famously the night before at Candle Bar, but this was something else. This was a full-on New York City I've-been-here-before flashback. I knew them. I had met them before.

Seven years prior on a Gay.com meet up, similar to the one the night before in the Upper West Side, we met at Oscar Wilde's for drinks and some laughs that soon after vanished into The City; a victim of the Razor Phone and continuously losing them. Here they were. This couple I had met so long ago, and really liked, and hoped, for the sake of proxy to our destination, they felt similarly of me.

We pulled into the gravel drive up to register our campsite and vehicle. My heart was racing, worrying that I'd flip out about being naked in front of a camp full of strangers, and once these guys discovered that they had met me before what they would do? The idea of the crazed murderers re-centralized itself in my imagination. I proceeded with caution as to the best time and place to tell them. Maybe I didn't have to? Not while we were setting up tarps and canopies, not while we were loading the unpacked trunk up with firewood, not while we were building a fire, but perhaps after three rounds of Fireball shots?

"NO FUCKING WAY! JOJO! JOJO!"

Fleetwood came bolting out from behind the cabin where he and I were peeing in the bushes together. I figured the most non-threatening time to tell them my secret was naked and peeing after the burn of the shots wore off.

"NO FUCKING WAY!"

JoJo couldn't believe it either. Snickers was confused and just sat on the picnic bench straddling the wood, resting his wood on the wood sucking on a beer. The safety in the reunion made me feel better about being stark naked in the middle of nowhere, and in telling them so, we ventured down to the pool. The big scary pool where I wasn't sure I was ready to be.

The four of us on the camp site had spent the last few hours getting acquainted, and I was comfortable to hang out, very literally hang out, around our site with them naked, but a few hundred people or so? Visions of middle school and being prodded for being the fat kid piled on top of the voice of Dr. Molina, "THAT'S YOU?" That was piling on top of my overall general appearance, and dysfunctions of late, and the chemo, and cancer, and career, and new boyfriend, and work, and money, and before I knew it, I was in the water.

Nothing had happened. No pointing and laughing, no gasps or stares at the body I was still adjusting to, just calm and quiet and non-threatening musical stylings of Gaga and Whitney. I looked around at the group of us, perched on the front corner of the pool by the steps, and noticed the beautiful rainbow of diversity in body shapes and sizes. Skin, so much skin, slick and kissed with the sun that had hair, and tattoos, and piercings, abnormalities, beautiful flaws. The laughter, and smiling, and camaraderie that rumbled over the blare of the speakers seemed to exude an air of don't-give-a-fuck-ness that I wanted to tap into. I took notes.

Sun chairs laden with men who were overweight, underweight, had dadbods, were muscle bound, thick, thin, white, gold, brown, black, tall, short, single, married, widowed, coiffed, bald, bearded, clean shaven. I began to slowly recognize through the forming fog of vodka-lemonade and my aviators that this was a safe space, an escape. Maybe I'd never look like the sunbathing slabs with the impossibly technically good physiques. Maybe I looked more like the men who were thicker in sections not often viewed as acceptable, but no one there was offensive to me, and it seemed as if that was a common thread as I watched odd pairings of a community I belonged to interact, and celebrate themselves, and each other.

New was this feeling I was watching unfold in front of me, the excitement of coming to terms and reckoning with myself through an event I was so apprehensive about approaching. Quietly, I laughed to myself as I spread my arms across the concrete side of the pool, still in the water, leaning my head back towards the sun. It now seemed too silly that I hid for all those months, hid during a time when I needed the most support, care, and attention. Unsure how I could not have understood at the time that acceptance was out there; I was bathing in a pool of it.

"Ed! Come on we're gonna play Chicken!"

Fleetwood snapped me out of my crunchy granola, feel-good realizations, and tried to hoist me up on his back; all two hundred and forty, not-quite-there, naked, unashamed pounds of me.

210 Seize the Day

Two Sound of Music's and a Moon Over Buffalo were left behind me as I approached Audition Season 2014 with a vigor that felt old hat at this point. I'd booked three shows back-to-back straight out the gate, not six months after my transplant, so it felt as though I was back and better than ever. Validated? But Audition Season came and went with underwhelming results, and I resigned myself to my desk job at a private arts club in the Upper East Side. I liked the job enough to allow the worm of doubt to creep in, and to question whether or not I'd be happier in a career in hospitality.

FINDING REASONS TO SMILE AGAIN. IN A HOT TUB. AT A MANSION. THAT WASN'T MINE. IN FLORIDA.

Shortly after Memphis had dumped me for a chorus boy he'd known for ten days in the Midwest, I dumped an offer that was handed to me from a theatre I had worked at the year before in Arizona: 'The Angry Housewives'. The script was.., the script was... written with words that were printed on a page, and I was about as excited to go do it as I was about cleaning the toilet at home. So, I was relieved to receive a phone call from a theatre, I'd completely forgotten I had contacted, offering me the role of Fred Graham in Kiss Me Kate, in Florida. There was no contest in arguing that this was a much better contract, a much better script, and much better music. Fred was a dream role, and even though I was fundamentally excited to be adding that name to my resume, part of me still didn't care. I should have been all 'booked and blessed' but I felt more like booked and bothered.

Being an actor had become a masturbatory malfunction, reflective of my self-displeasures at my two respective hospitals; should feel good, didn't feel good. The other side of the pancake wasn't cake at all and was proving to be a really fucking disorienting tightrope. On one side was familiar Musical Theatre. On the other side? Every other option. I found myself in another dark pit. I should have felt grateful to be alive. I should have felt however one feels when comparing the lacking aspects of their lives to surviving cancer. I should have let it all roll off my shoulders because, hey, I beat the Big C and I'm alive and well. I should have, but I

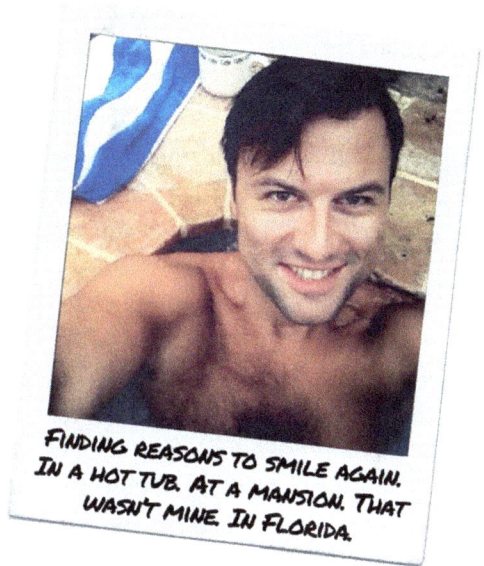

didn't, because I couldn't, because I didn't know how. So, at my place of employment in my dark suit, white shirt, and tie I'd sit at the big wooden desk in the big marble foyer greeting the big dressed up money that walked through the door for dinner and cocktails and felt so little. What was I doing? What was I accomplishing? Was the highlight of my performance career going to be eighteen weeks of Hairspray in Reno Again, I felt lost. Who is this new person? What does this new person that I seemingly am do?

"You wanna go see Newsies with me in an hour?"

No. I didn't. But I hadn't sat in a theatre in a long time and free tickets to anything on Broadway, especially something that's closing, is not something you say no to. So instead of spending another afternoon guzzling down frozen margaritas at Blockhead's in Midtown, I met Crutchie at the Nederlander for a matinee of tiny dancers and Disney. Maybe a show was what I needed? Maybe something to jump-start my motor? The last time I was even in the Nederlander Theatre was to see Rent for my sixteenth birthday. As we shuffled into the lobby, collecting our Playbills, we were directed to the second row in the orchestra all the way left. A quarter of the stage was missing from my line of sight, and a crick in my neck was already starting to pull as I gauged just how I was going to see the rest of the stage from my seat.

"Great, I'll miss half of it."

The murmur in the house went down with the lights as the conductor appeared to a smattering of applause. As the overture soared high above the balcony, kissing the ornate ceiling and walls of the old Broadway theatre, I could feel little hairline fractures start to form in the armor I'd placed over myself for the past eight months. The professional dry spell and lackluster excitement of what I had on deck, the breakup, the irregularity of a regular job had coated me in a layer of protective tin that was keeping my identity at bay.

Once the curtain was up and the cast appeared, these men, boys that were a quarter of my size leaped and bounded high above the stage floor. Sound came out of them that one would never expect from a person of that stature. Energy exuded from every limb cracking me across the face in a Christopher Gattelli wake up call. I fought the feelings that were welling up inside my chest; acting was selfish, auditioning was masturbatory, theatre was thankless, and empty. But not even halfway through act one, I found myself sitting in the red velvet seats weeping.

Trying to remain silent so as to not draw any unwanted attention, I was basically smothering an ugly cry into the Playbill. Had any one of the cast members seen me they would have thought that some crazy person was having an episode house left. They wouldn't have been entirely wrong.

Newsies is not a sad or emotionally havoc-wreaking show. But it wasn't about the show, it wasn't about me, it wasn't even about cancer. For every performance an actor does, there is someone, even if it's just one person in that audience that desperately needs what you're doing on that stage, whether they realize it or not. It's a ripple effect. The show is the pebble, and the audience is the lake. Once the pebble is thrown out into the lake, the effects it can have on those present can be minor or insurmountable. I was caught in that ripple. I had never made that connection or realization before and once the thought was coherent in my mind and the dots had been connected, I completely surrendered to the Newsies. I realized why I wanted to do all of this in the first place. I remembered why I loved this:

I was fourteen years old, and it was my second time in New York City. Times Square stank of urine, garbage, and pizza in the early summer's rich humidity. I was simultaneously hungry and nauseous, which I could not claim to be the first time that occurred. My two sisters, Crissy, and Jeanie, and Mother and Father, walked down the West side of Broadway en-route to the Ford Theatre on West 42nd Street. The few blocks between The Starlight Diner and the theatre had me sticky and drenched. It felt like someone had just sprayed me in the face with hot water from an aerosol can. Evidently, April in The City is no joke.

"Eddie, look out!"

I crossed 45th Street against the light. No cars were coming so I took it upon myself not to clog the sidewalk unnecessarily, and cross with pedestrian traffic. My parents, having not been to The City in nearly two decades, were being hypersensitive to every matter of safety, and rightfully so. The first time I was in The City was with Father's sister, Aunt Phyllis. We went to the top of the Statue of Liberty, and to Ellis Island. I had left my camera by the immigration wall where our families name is engraved and ran back to get it. Phyllis nearly had an aneurism.

"What? No one was coming!"

Even then I knew that to get to where you're going in New York, you have to keep up with the current. And besides, I was really fucking excited; we were about to see our first Broadway show: 42nd Street. Despite being involved in theatre in some capacity most of our lives, no one in the family had ever seen a show on Broadway before.

I consciously assessed that I didn't really understand the magnitude of what I was about to watch. Sure, I'd been listening to Broadway for years, an aficionado, if you asked me, but to actually be here in New York City, with a ticket in my pocket, I was struck nearly mute at the anticipation.

The line outside of the theatre was forever long, and an overwhelming impatience took over me; a worry that we were never going to get inside in time. Slowly shuffling along, through the sea of the corn-fed, we finally slinked towards the threshold to Mecca. The tallest man I had ever seen in my fourteen years of life extended his large hand towards me, beckoning for my ticket. It was an uncommon circumstance for me to be unevenly eye level with someone where I had to look up at a person and I stared. He ripped off the perforated stub and motioned for me to cross into the house. All I wanted to do was stand next to him and bask in his height, but I moved on with the flow of the line into the grand lobby and its mosaic and marble floor, lined with immense pillars.

Our seats were in the back of the orchestra. The shadow that the balcony cast over the red velvet seats on the main floor was eerie and imposing, exacerbated only by the old ornate theatre, the murals, the decorative molding. I sat on velvet; a luxury dampened by my swollen legs being squished together by the arm rests of the seat. I was a sizable fourteen-year-old.

Paging through the perfume and show advertisements in my official Broadway Playbill I searched for David Elder, Phyllis's new best friend. She handed her life as a public-school guidance counselor in for coin jackets and high waisted trousers. This was her Broadway debut; she, they had made it! After two hundred pages of Estee Lauder and Mamma Mia ads, I found his headshot, handsome and smirking back at me. My parts fluttered for a moment before my entire being sank into the floor.

"HOLY SHIT!"

Crissy turned to me and inquired what my sudden outburst was about.

"You guys! THE MOM FROM MY GIRL TWO IS IN THIS SHOW!!!!!"

My excitement escalated from pretty, to really fucking. This woman was the co-star of one of my favorite movies ever!

"No WAY!"

Everything went dark. Giggling with my sisters, I wriggled around a bit in the seat that my chubby body barely fit into, rolling my official Broadway Playbill into a tube in my hand. The first smattering of applause filled the room as the spotlight from somewhere in the heavens illuminated the top of someone's head at the foot of the stage. The conductor? Maybe it was an anniversary, or a birthday? They announced those kinds of things at the theatres I had performed in; that must have been it. All I saw was white light and the outline of the head in front of me.

The applause died down. In one jerking motion, the hand and baton of the conductor slammed itself downward and heavenly orchestrations broke through the silence of the huge hushed room. The overture soared above the heads of even the highest seats in the Mezzanine. I bellowed with excitement. The black and white keys cued the trumpets, granting permission for the glorious red curtain to rustle itself alive, and rise about three feet off the stage. Hovering above the floor, hundreds of pounds of velvet revealed a long line of beautiful legs; feet, clapping against the stage like a rainstorm. Stomping in rhythmic fits of style and specificity. The thunder of the tapping crushed my lungs as I sat there afraid to blink, afraid to miss a second. Needles and pins rushed over me, and I moved to the edge of my seat.

My heart leapt in my chest at the final stomp of the number and the screams and cheers of the theatre seekers egged on the cast of beautiful people for more. Their approval deafened any other sound in the room. It was the only sound that mattered. Still catching my breath from the thrill and pleasure of the first number, it suddenly felt like this show was trying to kill me. She appeared from stage right like an old friend you haven't laid eyes on for a long time and see in the grocery store, unsure if it's them. She floated to center stage in all white, clutch in hand, her blond hair curled and frizzed out from under her hat. It was her. The Mom from My Girl Two! It was Christine Ebersole. I couldn't take my eyes off her as she moved in a way that I'd only seen in the black and white movies Grandma used to make us watch when she was baby-sitting us as kids. I was freaking out.

I became unaware that my too-cool-for-school, angsty, adolescent front had completely dropped off. I was too busy looking as hard as I could at the 1930s flying in front of me in high-waisted pants, evening gowns, and shiny gold coined suits. The larger-than-life sets, unlike anything I had ever witnessed before, glided across the floor like a swan. How could humans move something so effortlessly? Effortlessly pivoting, entering and exiting through splashes of lights, lights in colors that I never thought could exist. The sets I was watching were dancing, sliding along the stage like they were on an ice rink. They had to be automated; they had to be tracked or something. Nothing moves that steadily.

Julian Marsh brandished Peggy Sawyer's yellow scarf in his hands with triumph and new life and shoved it into his pocket. The ear-splitting sound of cheers and applause replaced the sounds of LeDucas that had spent two-and-a-half glorious hours clamoring from wall to wall. I didn't want it to end. I could have sat there all day in this world that was created in front of me, lost to the city streets just on the other side of the theatre doors. Once again, the colorful, gorgeous cast of characters appeared for their curtain call. The applause swelled at each entrance and bow, leaving the few hundred of us in a void of hands repeatedly greeting each other, nearly unable to hear our own whoops and hollers.

The curtain fell for us one last time, like it was some kind of circus trick being bestowed upon us, the members of the audience. The house lights came up on the breathtaking theatre – I'd nearly forgotten where I was - and a murmur erupted from the crowd. The enthralled audience whom, to me, were now the attendees of the Ascott Opening Race collectively stood, ruffled their Playbills and Bloomingdale's shopping bags, and muddled their way back out into the sweltering Manhattan streets. But not us. The family stayed behind to be escorted by the house manager into the grand lobby of the theatre to meet Phyllis after the crowd dispersed. We stood behind the last row of the orchestra when a thin, bald man in all black, walked over and introduced himself and his agenda: Les.

Head to the lobby, meet Phyllis, go backstage. Backstage. That word hit me: I WAS GOING BACKSTAGE AT A BROADWAY SHOW AND MEETING A BROADWAY STAR!!!

The angst had painted itself back across my face as I tried to pretend that I wasn't leaping out of my skin at the prospect of the next fifteen minutes. Les lead us into the grand lobby, which emptied very quickly. Soon we were alone, just the family, standing on the comedy and tragedy mask mosaic in the marble floor waiting for Phyllis. She came out of nowhere, framed by her dark brown, choppy hair waving and squealing a "Hi" that had become quintessential to her visits. We snapped some photos of the family in the lobby before it was time.

Through the theatre, into the wings, down the windy stairs, and down the long hallways to the dressing rooms we passed more men and women in all black, some with pouches tied around their waists, others with clip boards and headsets. This was the busy underbelly to put a show together and make it tick and work. It hit me: Phyllis was one of them. She was one of the people that made an enormous and glorious Broadway show chug along. I walked a little taller down that hallway. I was proud to be there, and to be there with her.

"That's Ms. Ebersole's dressing room."

GASP! WHAT? Crissy, Jeanie, and I looked back and forth at each other, collectively whispering to Phyllis if we could meet her. Obviously since they worked together, they were friends. Of course we could meet her. Like a family portrait we arranged ourselves outside the door to receive 'The Mom from My Girl Two.' The door was ajar ever so slightly to where you could almost see a figure inside the dimly lit room. Phyllis timidly approached the door and knocked.

"Ms. Ebersole? Ms. Ebersole, my family is here and would love to meet you."

Suddenly the door flung open to a strikingly tall woman in full beat, wearing only a wig cap, her under garments, tights, and a smile. She stood inside the door by her make-up station in a bevel leaning gracefully over her lit-up mirror. There she was. I was staring; I was definitely staring and trying to play it cool and cordial.

"Hello."

My basement was completely flooded in a way that only an adolescent gay boy would understand. It seemed like we were standing there for hours before she came over and said hello, briskly shutting the door. Was she mad? How did the door open in the first place?

I don't even remember going to Mr. Elder's dressing room. I was lost in the Ebersole. She was so tall, so glamorous, even in her skivvies; I was completely enamored with her. What I do remember is the bus ride home where plans and plots began to form. Whatever it took, whatever I had to do to make it happen, I was going to be part of whatever it was that involved this glorious Glamazon and her massive lashes and wig cap.

The Newsies took their bows and I leapt to my feet masking my blubbering under the thunder of hands meeting throughout the audience. Crutchie looked up at me curiously wondering if I had completely snapped. I couldn't even look at him. I knew I'd fall even farther apart. I was so grateful to have been offered this ticket, this opportunity to rediscover what I loved. Having been lost for nearly two years without really realizing the location of my compass, I'd just been going through the motions of post-cancer life. I'd been defaulting to what I knew (auditions, gym, work) without really focusing on a goal, or end point, or destination, or really anything other than going through the motions. But here it was, my compass, applauding, and bowing, and living on stage. I found me again, behind the walls of the Nederlander Theatre. The magic of Disney and the cast of Newsies saved me.

Crutchie and I walked out of the theatre. Without saying a word, we walked down the block towards Eighth Avenue until I stopped Crutchie right outside of Dean and Deluca.

"You don't even know what that show just did for me. Thank you!"

We separated, heading toward and boarding our respective trains home. Over the hurdle of uncontrollable wailing, there was now a heavy fire and pit burning in my gut. The kind that makes you want to run a marathon, invincibly doing so with ease. I leapt out of the 72nd Street train station like a real, really oversized Newsie and booked it up to my apartment. I dove onto my desk chair and pulled the script of Kiss Me Kate out of the drawer I had placed it in figuring I would get to it when I felt like it. I felt like it. I grabbed a yellow highlighter and took the script to task, illustrating the magnitude of material I was going to be painting onto my brain.

Hacking my way through bastardized Shakespeare, I deterred for a moment and began to seek out the cast on social media. Nearly immediately, I found the Newsie who won most of my attention and opened a messenger window.

"I spent the majority of this year frustrated with this business (the theatre) and uncertain if I wanted to stay in it. I was looking for other options to leave and redirect myself towards something else. I stopped auditioning for a few months; I shut down. I wasn't happy. Today I saw Newsies for the first time, and sat there, in probably the worse seats ever, but it didn't matter, with tears running down my face. Your cast living their lives on stage putting 3000% into the show was so refreshing and inspiring and enchanting to watch. I was and still am in awe of you all. I had a very specific moment where I just involuntarily thought 'I love this. I wanted to do this for the rest of my life.' It was at that moment that all of the times I thought of leaving the business because it felt selfish and masturbatory and shallow, vanished because I realized that someone in any audience, someone like me, could be moved, touched, inspired, and changed because of what was happening on stage.

Now I have a show booked, but I wasn't anything more than fundamentally excited for it until today. I can't wait for rehearsals. You and your company are responsible for that. You have completely changed my perspective on my career and kind of my life as a whole, to the point where every time I walk into an audition

I'm going to think 'give them Newsies.' You are all amazing. I cannot thank you enough. You saved me today."

I felt absolutely stupid sending the message, fan-girling all over a Newsie, but from the emotional firework that had been set off inside The Nederlander Theatre, a sense of invincibility had come over me. For the first time since I'd been discharged from Sloan Kettering nearly two years prior, I felt as though I had cast an anchor and could stand confidently in what I was doing. Why it had taken me two years was beyond my comprehension. Why it took a stage of 5'6" and under dancers leaping through the air, weightless, belting their big dancer asses off is beyond me. What I do know, is that the day I saw Newsies was the day I decided that musical theatre could, in fact, save lives, because it saved mine.

Edward Miskie

People Like Us - The Epilogue

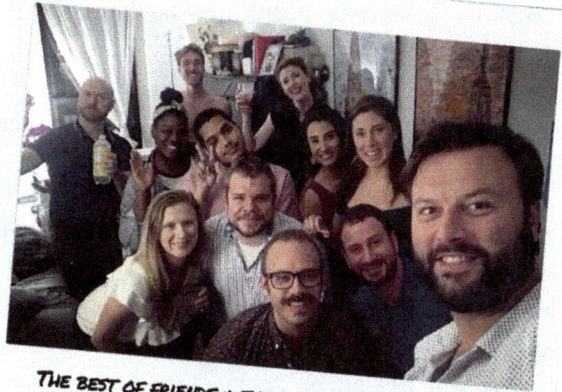

THE BEST OF FRIENDS + THE BEST OF TIMES IN MY TINY LITTLE APARTMENT ON WEST 73RD STREET.

See? Told ya. Cancer is really fucking terrible. And if you thought that was bad, know that I didn't even go into the blood transfusions, or the platelet transfusions. I didn't go into detail about being quarantined for five days because of a parasite I'd gotten from swimming in the Atlantic Ocean, or how I lost fifteen pounds in four days from excreting black and green water out of my body with a fever of 104. I never talked about Mother's five-hour run-around in the sweltering July summer to various uncommunicative Medicaid offices that nearly gave her a heart attack. I didn't even touch on the house call from public assistance, making sure I wasn't lying about having cancer, and working the system. I didn't talk about how I had to kick that social worker out of my apartment because, even having looked at me, very clearly being a cancer patient, he still harassed me, and asked very personal, unrelated questions. Though worth mentioning, I didn't discuss the disability office telling me to 'just make less than X amount' so that I could continue collecting full benefits. It made me wonder who's working which system? And finally, I didn't detail the funeral arrangements; cremated, and buried in one of those tree-pod things in my parent's backyard in Central Pennsylvania.

By all things medical and scientific I shouldn't be alive. My case, I'm told, is the baseline at Sloan Kettering for all new cases of the same cancer I had, which is fucking scary. That means that should Seymour ever decide to return; my case is the source case for treatment. The day Dr. Anthony told me that I kind of barf smiled and exclaimed 'Wow!' But really, I meant, 'Oh shit, I really wish you hadn't told me that.' I try to focus on the fact that the countering side of this information is that because of my case, others are being helped. There is balance.

Beating cancer is amazing. Every time you choose to out yourself to someone as a cancer survivor, they'll remind you of how amazing it is, and you should never shortchange yourself that feat, ever. Don't let anyone ever bring you down from that because as a survivor, people, maybe those you thought were friends, maybe those you just knew peripherally, will say some weird, and fucked up shit to you. My favorites?

Someone from my Hairspray cast told everyone that I was lying about having cancer, and that it was actually AIDS.

A former co-worker, who got upset that I told the 'wrong person' I knew him, told me, "I hope it comes back and you don't win this time".

And my personal favorite was an acting coach and director in NYC, whom I had been friends with for years, asked me, "So now that your cancer's gone, how are you going to get men to sleep with you?"

Silence will, as well, be strange. Like Beadle, who brushed the whole thing off, you'll be left behind by those who can't handle, don't want to handle, or don't know how to handle your circumstances. And that's okay! Those who matter will rise to the top. You will know who your true friends are, and that's an incredible feeling.

But as amazing as it is that you're on the other side of the hardest thing you've ever had to overcome, survivorship is equally as scary as treatment, maybe worse, maybe just different. No, living to see another day is not awful, and you should be grateful for each sunrise you're afforded, but with that said, alongside of your newfound freedom and release from hospital life, you have a new leash. You have a leash, which I call 'the fear spiral', also known as PTSD!

What, you may ask, is 'the fear spiral'?

Well!

"Why is this cut taking more than a few days to heal? Why do I have a headache on only one side of my head? What is this ache in my side? Why does my stomach hurt? What if this sore throat turns into esophageal cancer and I die; or worse yet, live and have to eat out of a feeding tube for the rest of my depleted life? Is breathing difficult right now or is that just because I'm at the gym? What is this bump on my head? Where did that bruise come from? Why haven't I noticed that before? What if it comes back? What if I have to go back? Don't make me go back. If I go back, I'm not going to live. I'm going to die. I'm definitely going to die. Am I dying right now? Why am I sweating? Were the transplant graphs being rejected? Was my immune system failing? Is this death? I should call my parents cause I'm dying."

That, ladies, gents, and whom-so-ever you identify yourself as, is the fear spiral. The panic and anxiety that you are, or will, die from the slightest ailment is onset nearly immediately upon release from your hospital of choice. Maybe you've had this before your final discharge, maybe you haven't, but it's coming.

Each cut or bruise that I accrued was monitored like a government secret to make sure it healed in, what I considered to be, a timely manner, lest I obviously had developed Leukemia and would shortly die. Similarly, to a friend's partner who was in a car accident, whose bruises didn't heal after a few weeks. He went to the hospital to have them checked and was dead before Christmas because of a Leukemia he had developed. I took that on and watched my bruises almost as compulsively as I checked Seymour. You become an absolute crazy hypochondriac person. You call the hospital and your doctors and try to diagnose whatever ailment it is that you think you have that's a preamble to what's sure to be the imminent end of your life. Sometimes you call your mom, or dad. My poor parents! The stupid shit I would subject them to was often so explainable, and not even remotely rational, but that's the fear spiral. That's how it goes.

Phantom pains, reminiscent to your ailment, will crawl all over your body. They throw you into a fissure so deep, and dark, and crippling that any sort of distraction will suffice no matter how self-destructive that distraction may be. The PTSD button becomes an involuntary friend paralyzing you at the notion or thought that it's back! It's growing!

Through all of this, you do your best to do whatever you can to stay on the straight-ish and narrow-ish. I became so concerned about what I was eating and the effects it may have on my body, grocery shopping became a conspiracy; the food against me. I started watching food and health documentaries on Netflix, which of course sent me into another spiral downward. I started actually reading labels on food products, which in the long run was good, but at the time was a nightmare. Anything unpronounceable went back on the shelves because obviously that was going to give me immediate cancer.

THANKS NETFLIX!

To exacerbate the documentaries, for out-patient, Sloan provided me with a nutritionist, email, and phone number. My nutritionist was cool as fuck with the level of patience and genuine understanding she had for my craziness. I had her email on VIP, and I sent her messages like I needed her permission to breath.

"Can I eat this?"

"Can I eat that?"

"Are these ingredients ok?"

"Will this re-trigger my cancer?"

If she didn't answer by the end of the day, I'd make sure that I called her line to follow up, making sure that she'd received my email.

There wasn't a single circumstance that I couldn't artfully turn into a death panel, and the littlest things would trigger it. The reality is nothing; the residual PTSD makes it nuclear. Cancer, and its aftershocks and tremors of surviving, look a hell of a lot like a post-war mental mine field. One false step, and your whole day, mood, and psyche are blown to bits.

I purposefully covered sex, dating, and body in this book, and not just for the sake of talking about it, but because I felt that, above most, in regard to cancer patients, it's not covered. Like my middle school sex-ed class where the curriculum was:

"Here's a penis. Here's a vagina. They make babies. Now we are going to watch 'Philadelphia'."

More needs to be said. I definitely should not have been lining up amusement park rides for the band-aid of my psyche. That's fucking dangerous under such circumstances. But I didn't stop being human, I didn't stop feeling, and needing, and wanting, and I didn't know how to translate normal human behavior into cancer patient terms. Evidently, no one else did either, because it wasn't discussed. I still don't have an answer for that.

I semi-continued my sex and dating life as I would have, had I not been a cancer patient. Especially after the fear of being alone post-Valentine-break-up really set in. I was on those apps day in and day out. Even now, I'll open someone's profile to find that we'd spoken sometime in 2012, and see said conversation in the present day, knowing then I was a patient, no bueno. That probably wasn't the best, but someone somewhere put a high price on dating and getting laid, and under my stubborn refusal to be a sick person, I still played into that. Even when my equipment wouldn't work, a plight I felt lasted entirely too long, and no one discussed with me, nor did I think/want to ask. I continued to attempt to make efforts at using it - and failed. And even though I gained great friends out of those app conversations and meetings (Senex, Big Daddy-J), in hindsight, it was more damaging than helpful.

Therapy helped for a while. Dr. Aurora did her job as long as she could, or as long as I'd let her. I'm still unsure which is more accurate. She would poke and prod at me, forcing cultivation and change, until she was just prodding the same things week after week. She would sit there and stare at me, calculating how much hair had grown back since last I saw her, and how much muscle tone was starting to reappear on my post-transplant skeleton. She'd listen to everything I was saying, but not forging forward, as she had before, as if she were bored.

"So, you're scared that everything you physically feel is going to lead to cancer. How does that make you feel?"

I JUST TOLD YOU AND THAT'S EXACTLY WHAT I JUST SAID!

Her overstuffed sofa wasn't comfortable anymore. I began to judge her matronly wardrobe out of frustration of her paraphrase therapy. More and more it began to feel as though I was going to a therapy session with Siri on my iPhone, and Siri was free. So, I stopped. I left her office and never went back.

It's a rocky road forward. Sadly, not like the ice cream, but once you get some footing of your day to day, you can start figuring yourself out again, and it gets better. Going back to your old normal is nearly impossible, I've found; I've come close, but haven't gotten there, nor am I sure I'd want to. I'm arguably a better person than I was before. I have a better attitude, and a hunger for life that I didn't even know was there. I've learned how to pick my battles, and recognize what's important, and what isn't. Family is important, chosen or otherwise. But I still struggle, I still spiral, less often than not, but it still happens. Sense memory will still kick me down a few pegs.

The smell of hand sanitizer takes me a few seconds to overcome, being reminded of the thick stench of the dispensers in every room of every hospital. To me, that is what death and sadness smells like, hand sanitizer.

When all is said and done, you've still beat cancer. You're still alive. You've been afforded a really beautiful, scary chance to pull a Madonna and reinvent yourself however you'd like. Start from scratch, be a better human, live your life like you wouldn't or couldn't before. Throw caution to the wind. Go places, do things, and meet people you wouldn't normally. Personally, I'm obsessed with the idea of showing up to an airport, asking what the next departing flight is, and buying a last-minute ticket; just go. Go on adventures. Be a tourist wherever you are, unabashedly so, and see everything. Take pictures, hug everyone, tell everyone you love them, empty your savings, do whatever the fuck you want with it, and don't feel badly about your choices afterwards.

This book was a passion project I wrote to help people by talking about some things that I was embarrassed about during and after treatment. I wanted to bring up the tough stuff so that it wouldn't be tough anymore; learn from my fuck ups and missteps.

Along the road I've met other survivors who've been an inspiration not only to me, but also in my writing. We've learned from each other. And whereas I hope that you, as the reader, have been helped immensely through either laughter, insight, example, or camaraderie, I sincerely hope, that as wonderful of a journey as this has been, and as awful of a journey that this has been, we all can rebuild from having been torn down.

Remember: Eat. Laugh. Leave.

"You are braver than you believe, stronger than you seem, and smarter than you think." - Winnie The Pooh, A. A. Milne.

Bibliography, References & Credit Lexicon

The Cast:
Edward Miskie - Musical of Life; based on self © 1986

Seymour, Dr. Orin, Nurse Audrey, Chiffon, Ronette, Crystal, Seymour - Little Shop of Horrors; Little Shop of Horrors; music by Alan Menken and Howard Ashman, book by Howard Ashman based on the 1960 film of the same name. © 1982

FINAL DRAFT IN HAND FOR THE FIRST RUN OF MY BADASS BOOK (APRIL 2017)

Mother, Father, - Ragtime; book by Terrence McNally, lyrics by Lynn Ahrens, and music by Stephen Flaherty © 1996

Dr. Turner, Dr. Zack, Dr. Richie, Cassie - A Chorus Line; music by Marvin Hamlisch, lyrics by Edward Kleban and book by James Kirkwood, Jr. and Nicholas Dante © 1975

Dr. Mame Anthony, Gooch, Vera, Dr. Beauregard - Mame; book by Jerome Lawrence and Robert Edwin Lee, music and lyrics by Jerry Herman © 1966

Dr. Deuteronomy, Grizabella, Jennyanydots, RumTum Gus - Cats; musical by Andrew Lloyd Webber, based on Old Possum's Book of Practical Cats by T. S. Eliot © 1980

Anthony, Beadle, Turpin - Sweeney Todd; music and lyrics by Stephen Sondheim, book by Hugh Wheeler, based on the 1973 play Sweeney Todd, the Demon Barber of Fleet Street by Christopher Bond © 1979

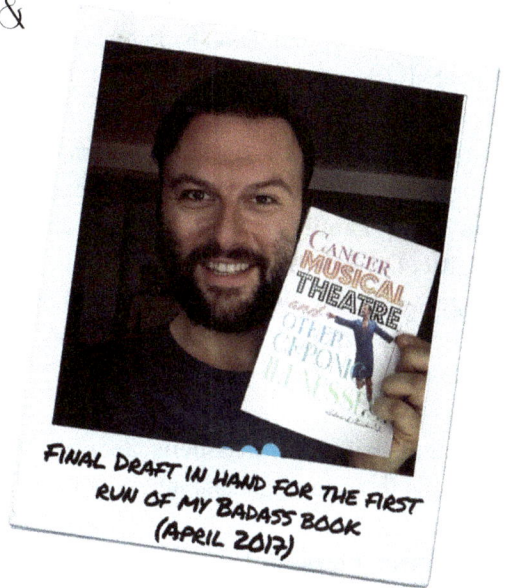

Myrrhine, Nurse Lampito, Nurse Cleonice, Nurse Robin - Lysistrata Jones; music by Lewis Flinn, book by Douglas Carter Beane, adaptation of Aristophanes' comedy Lysistrata © 2011

Nurse Dot, Nurse Blaire, Nurse Harriet - Sunday in The Park with George; music and lyrics by Stephen Sondheim and book by James Lapine © 1984 **Von Trapp Family Doctors, Dr. Max, Dr. Liesel, Dr. Marta, Dr. Gretle, Dr. Brigitte, Dr. Friedrich, Nurse Elsa** - The Sound of Music; music by Richard Rodgers, lyrics by Oscar Hammerstein II, book by Howard Lindsay and Russel Crouse on the memoir of Maria von Trapp, The Story of the Trapp Family Singers © 1959

Claude, Berger, Dionne, Sheila, Jeanine, Woof - Hair; book and lyrics by James Rado and Gerome Ragni and music by Galt MacDermot © 1967

Alan, Dean, Lizzie, Sakarian, Arlene - Baby; music by David Shire, lyrics by Richard Maltby, book by Sybille Pearson, based on a story developed by Susan Yankowitz © 1983

Dr. Flynn, Nurse Morton, Nurse Roxy, Nurse Velma, Ms. Sunshine - Chicago; music by John Kander, lyrics by Fred Ebb, book by Ebb and Bob Fosse © 1975

Dr. Aurora, Dr. Molina, Valentine, Marcos, Warnden, Esteban, Marta, Orderlies - Kiss of The Spider Woman; music by John Kander and Fred Ebb, book by Terrence McNally, based on the Manuel Puig novel El Beso de la Mujer Araña © 1990

Yonkers, Toreadorables - Gypsy; music by Jule Styne, lyrics by Stephen Sondheim, and a book by Arthur Laurents © 1959

Doralee - 9 To 5; music and lyrics by Dolly Parton, book by Patricia Resnick, based on the screenplay by Resnick and Colin Higgins © 2008.

Dr. Marvin, Dr. Whizzer - Falsettos; book by James Lapine and William Finn, music and lyrics by William Finn © 1992

Nurse Wyndham - Legally Blonde; music and lyrics by Laurence O'Keefe and Nell Benjamin, book by Heather Hach; based on the novel Legally Blonde by Amanda Brown and the 2001 film © 2001, 2007

Nurse Yvonne, Nurse Yvette, Nurse Kim, Dr. Tam, Dr. Chris, Thuy - Miss Saigon; music by Claude-Michel Schönberg and Alain Boublil, lyrics by Boublil and Richard Maltby, Jr © 1989
Nurse Trix - Drowsy Chaperone; musical with book by Bob Martin and Don McKellar and music and lyrics by Lisa Lambert and Greg Morrison © 1998

Dr. Gloriosus, Nurse Philia, Senex, Hero, Phila - A Funny Thing Happened on The Way to The Forum; music and lyrics by Stephen Sondheim and book by Burt Shevelove and Larry Gelbart © 1962

Jojo, Fleetwood, Snickers, Slick, Memphis - The Life; book by David Newman, Ira Gasman and Cy Coleman, music by Coleman, lyrics by Gasman © 1990

Crutchie - Newsies; music by Alan Menken, lyrics by Jack Feldman, book by Harvey Fierstein © 2011

Drood - The Mystery of Edwin Drood; written by Rupert Holmes based on the unfinished Charles Dickens novel The Mystery of Edwin Drood © 1985

Bruce Bogtrotter - Matilda; music and lyrics by Tim Minchin, adapted by Anthony Kelly, based on the children's book by Roald Dahl © 2010

Table of Contents
References & Credits

ACT I

Where Am I Now? - Lysistrata Jones; music by Lewis Flinn, book by Douglas Carter Beane, adaptation of Aristophanes' comedy Lysistrata © 2011

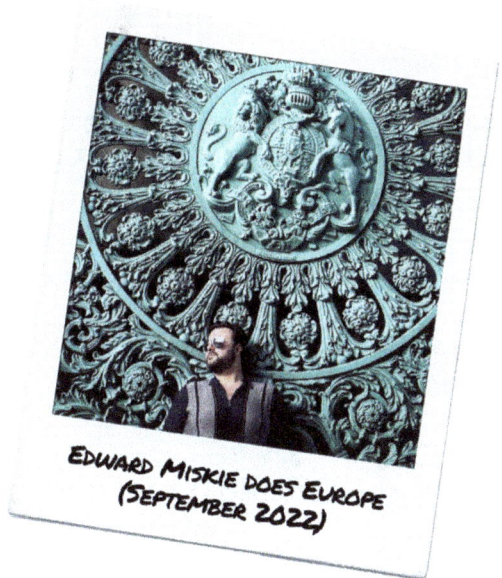

EDWARD MISKIE DOES EUROPE (SEPTEMBER 2022)

Jellicle Ball - Cats; composed by Andrew Lloyd Webber, based on Old Possum's Book of Practical Cats by T. S. Eliot © 1980

A Sweet Little Guy Named Seymour - Little Shop of Horrors; music by Alan Menken and Howard Ashman, book by Howard Ashman based on the 1960 film of the same name. © 1982

Park & 73rd - A Chorus Line; music by Marvin Hamlisch, lyrics by Edward Kleban and a book by James Kirkwood, Jr. and Nicholas Dante © 1975

The Barricade - Les Misérables; music by Claude-Michel Schonberg, book and lyrics by Alain Boublil, Jean-Marc Natel, and Herbert Kretzmer © 1980

The Worst Pies in London - Sweeney Todd; music and lyrics by Stephen Sondheim, book by Hugh Wheeler based on the Christopher Bond play Sweeney Todd: The Demon Barber of Fleet Street © 1979

Finishing The Hat - Sunday in The Park with George; music and lyrics by Stephen Sondheim and book by James Lapine. The musical was inspired by the painting A Sunday Afternoon on the Island of La Grande Jatte by Georges Seurat © 1984

What Is It You Cunt Face? - The Sound of Music (ish); music by Richard Rodgers, lyrics by Oscar Hammerstein II, book by Howard Lindsay and Russel

Crouse on the memoir of Maria von Trapp, The Story of the Trapp Family Singers © 1959

Shining, Gleaming, Streaming, Flaxen, Waxen - Hair; book and lyrics by James Rado and Gerome Ragni and music by Galt MacDermot © 1967

Poor Jerusalem - Jesus Christ Superstar; music by Andrew Lloyd Webber and lyrics by Tim Rice © 1970

The Old Razzle Dazzle - Chicago; music by John Kander, lyrics by Fred Ebb, book by Fred Ebb and Bob Fosse © 1975

Baby - book by Sybille Pearson, based on a story developed with Susan Yankowitz, music by David Shire, and lyrics by Richard Maltby, Jr. © 1983

Everything's Coming Up Roses - Gypsy; music by Jule Styne, lyrics by Stephen Sondheim, and a book by Arthur Laurents © 1959

Over the Wall - Kiss of the Spider Woman; music by John Kander and Fred Ebb, book by Terrence McNally, based on the novel El Beso de la Mujer Araña by Manuel Puig; © 1990

Get Out & Stay Out - 9 to 5; music and lyrics by Dolly Parton. It features a book by Patricia Resnick, based on the screenplay by Resnick and Colin Higgins © 2008

ACT II

It's Today - Mame; Mame; book by Jerome Lawrence and Robert Edwin Lee, music and lyrics by Jerry Herman © 1966

Waving Through a Window - Dear Evan Hansen; music by Pasek and Paul, book by Steven Levenson © 2015

This Had Better Stop - Falsettos; book by James Lapine and William Finn, music and lyrics by William Finn © 1992

The Bend and Snap - Legally Blonde; music and lyrics by Laurence O'Keefe and Nell Benjamin, book by Heather Hach; based on the novel Legally Blonde by Amanda Brown and the 2001 film © 2001, 2007

Why, God - Miss Saigon; music by Claude-Michel Schönberg and Alain Boublil, lyrics by Boublil and Richard Maltby, Jr © 1989

Man In Chair - Drowsy Chaperone; musical with book by Bob Martin and Don McKellar and music and lyrics by Lisa Lambert and Greg Morrison © 1998

I'm Calm - A Funny Thing Happened on The Way to The Forum; music and lyrics by Stephen Sondheim and book by Burt Shevelove and Larry Gelbart © 1962

Three Little Words - Ghost the Musical; book and lyrics by Bruce Joel Rubin, music and lyrics by Dave Stewart and Glen Ballard © 2011, 1990

Regretful-Happy – Company; based on a book by George Furth with music and lyrics by Stephen Sondheim © 1970

Where There Never Was a Hat - Sunday in The Park with George; music and lyrics by Stephen Sondheim and book by James Lapine. The musical was inspired by the painting A Sunday Afternoon on the Island of La Grande Jatte by Georges Seurat © 1984

I'm Still Here - Follies; music and lyrics by Stephen Sondheim and a book by James Goldman © 1971

Into The Woods & Out of The Woods, The Steps of The Palace, Agony, The Greens - music and lyrics by Stephen Sondheim and book by James Lapine. The musical intertwines the plots of several Brothers Grimm and Charles Perrault fairy tales © 1986

Ladies And Their Sensitivities - Sweeney Todd; music and lyrics by Stephen Sondheim, book by Hugh Wheeler, based on the 1973 play Sweeney Todd, the Demon Barber of Fleet Street by Christopher Bond © 1979

My Body Is My Business - The Life; book by David Newman, Ira Gasman and Cy Coleman, music by Coleman, lyrics by Gasman © 1990

Seize The Day - Newsies; music by Alan Menken, lyrics by Jack Feldman, book by Harvey Fierstein © 2011

People Like Us - Leap of Faith; music by Alan Menken, lyrics by Glenn Slater, book by Janus Cercone and Slater © 2010

Additional Photos

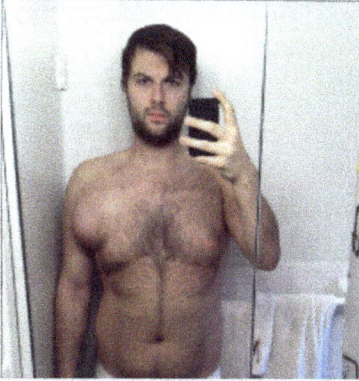

BATHROOM SELFIE BEFORE LEAVING
FOR DAY 1 OF CHEMO
(DECEMBER 2011)

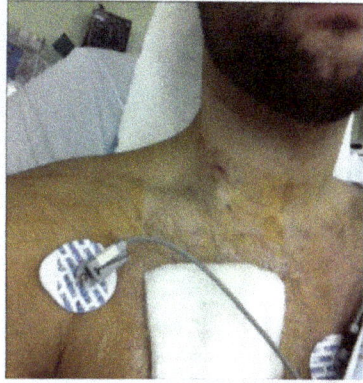

IMMEDIATELY AFTER PORT-
INSTALLATION SURGERY
(DECEMBER 2011)

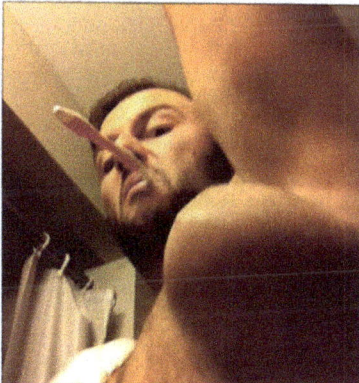

BEFORE CHEMO ROUND 1 WAS
FINISHED, SEYMOUR HAD GROWN
BACK, AND FAST (DECEMBER 2011)

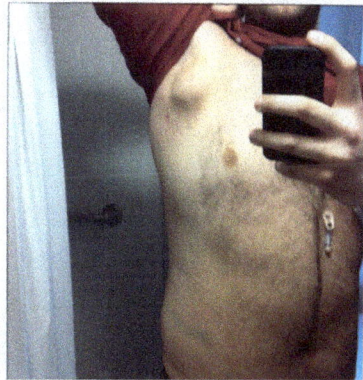

SEYMOUR AFTER CHEMO ROUND 2 -
SLIGHTLY SMALLER THAN BEFORE
(JANUARY 2012)

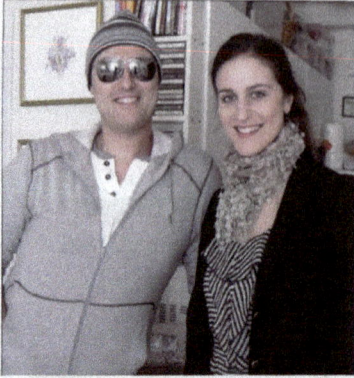

My sister & I at my Aunt's apartment in the Upper West Side (February 2012)

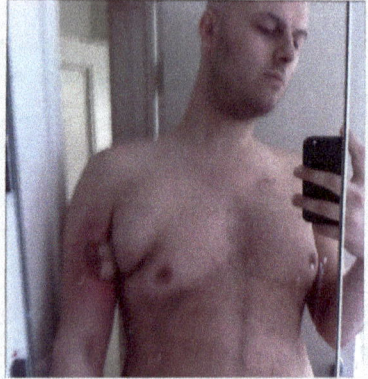

During Chemo Round 3, I got a staph infection & Seymour was bigger than ever (February 2012)

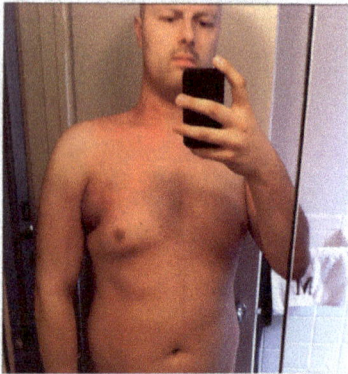

So-Long Chemo - bring on the radiation. (March 2012)

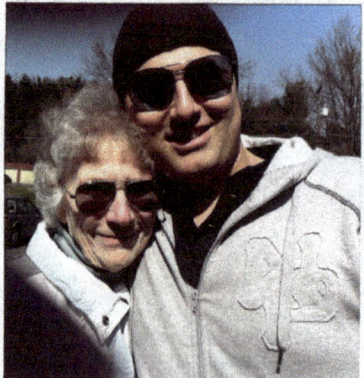

Visiting w/ my Maternal Grandmother in Central Pennsylvania on one of many visits home (March 2012)

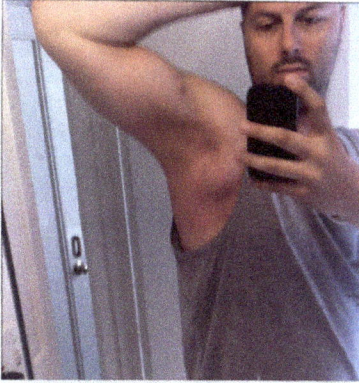

Seymour finally shrank permanently as my skin healed from Radiation (April 2012)

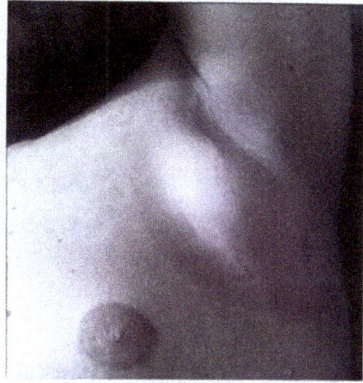

Healing little by little & Seymour is finally dying (April 2012)

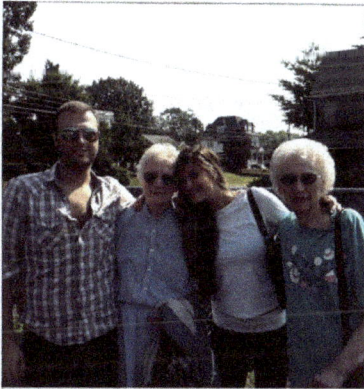

Brunch with my Grandmother, Mom, and Great Aunt Anna (May 2012)

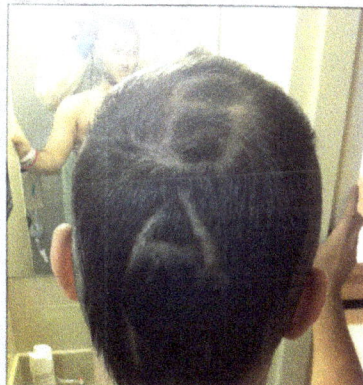

"Grizabella's" initials shaved onto my scalp (July 2012)

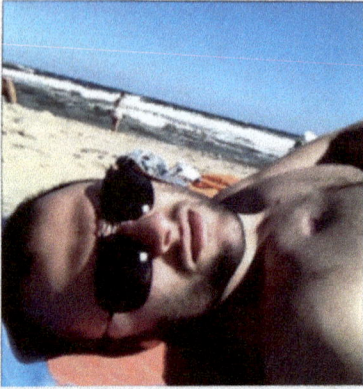

My trip to visit Violet in Florida
(November 2012)

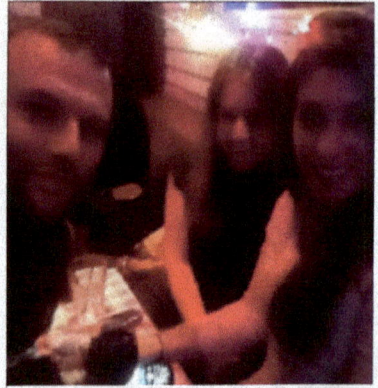

At Grizabella's bar in the Upper
West Side (November 2012)

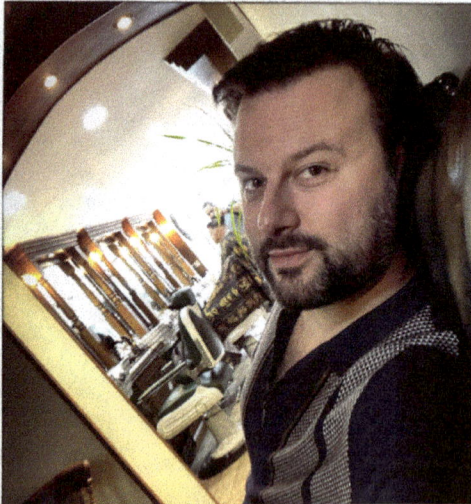

Shave & a Hair Cut – Two Bits!
Europe, September 2022

www.ingramcontent.com/pod-product-compliance
Lightning Source LLC
Chambersburg PA
CBHW062127020426
42335CB00013B/1124